NCCN Guidelines for Patients®

The essential guide for people facing cancer.

Based on care recommendations from leading cancer experts.

Explains high-quality cancer care provided at state-of-the-art cancer centers.

Reviewed and revised every year.

Did you know that top cancer centers across the United States work together to improve cancer care? This alliance of leading cancer centers is called the National Comprehensive Cancer Network® (NCCN®).

Because cancer care is always evolving, NCCN develops and frequently updates evidence-based cancer care recommendations used by health care providers worldwide. These recommendations are known as the NCCN Clinical Practice Guidelines in Oncology (NCCN Guidelines®).

The NCCN Guidelines for Patients plainly explain these expert recommendations, so you can talk with your care team about the best care for you.

These NCCN Guidelines for Patients are based on the NCCN Guidelines® for B-Cell Lymphomas, Version 4.2026 — May 20, 2026.

View the NCCN Guidelines for Patients free online: NCCN.org/patientguidelines

Find an NCCN Cancer Center near you: NCCN.org/cancercenters

Learn how the NCCN Guidelines for Patients are developed: NCCN.org/patient-guidelines-process

Connect with us

@NCCNorg @NCCNVideo NCCN @NCCNorg

Supporters

NATIONAL COMPREHENSIVE CANCER NETWORK®
NCCN FOUNDATION
Guiding Treatment. Changing Lives.

NCCN Guidelines for Patients are supported by funding from the NCCN Foundation®

NCCN Foundation gratefully acknowledges the following corporate supporters for helping to make available these NCCN Guidelines for Patients: AstraZeneca; Genentech, Inc.; and Genmab US, Inc.

NCCN independently adapts, updates, and hosts the NCCN Guidelines for Patients. Our corporate supporters do not participate in the development of the NCCN Guidelines for Patients and are not responsible for the content and recommendations contained therein.

To make a gift, visit
NCCNFoundation.org/Donate

To learn more, visit online
NCCN.org/patientguidelines
or email
PatientGuidelines@NCCN.org

Contents

NCCN Foundation seeks to support the millions of patients and their families affected by a cancer diagnosis by funding and distributing NCCN Guidelines for Patients. NCCN Foundation is also committed to advancing cancer treatment by funding the nation's promising doctors at the center of innovation in cancer research. For more details and the full library of patient and caregiver resources, visit NCCN.org/patients.

National Comprehensive Cancer Network (NCCN) and NCCN Foundation
3025 Chemical Road, Suite 100, Plymouth Meeting, PA 19462 USA

1 About follicular lymphoma

Follicular lymphoma (FL) develops from B lymphocytes, a type of white blood cell. In FL, excess numbers of abnormal B lymphocytes form clusters (follicles) in the lymph nodes and sometimes other tissues. It's a slow-growing lymphoma that doesn't always need treatment right away. Read this guide to learn more about the types of FL and how they're treated.

What is follicular lymphoma?

Follicular lymphoma (FL) is a blood cancer of lymphocytes. Lymphocytes are a type of white blood cell that helps fight and prevent infection. They are found in blood, lymph vessels, lymph nodes, and every organ in the body. Lymphocytes normally grow in response to infection or inflammation. When they grow on their own without proper regulation, they can develop into lymphoma like FL.

Types of lymphocytes

FL is a type of non-Hodgkin lymphoma (NHL). NHLs can develop from any type of lymphocytes, but B-cell lymphomas are the most common. There are many types of B-cell lymphomas. FL is 1 type.

There are 3 main types of lymphocytes:

- **B lymphocytes, or B cells**, make antibodies and eventually mature into plasma cells. An antibody is a protein that specifically targets infections or cancer cells and recruits other parts of the immune system.
- **T lymphocytes, or T cells**, help fight infections and cancer, and control immune responses.
- **Natural killer (NK) cells** can kill tumor cells or virus-infected cells.

Germinal centers

Follicular lymphoma (FL) starts in the temporary germinal centers of lymph nodes. These germinal centers are short-lived structures that form in response to infection or inflammation. When B cells within germinal centers grow out of control, they can develop into FL.

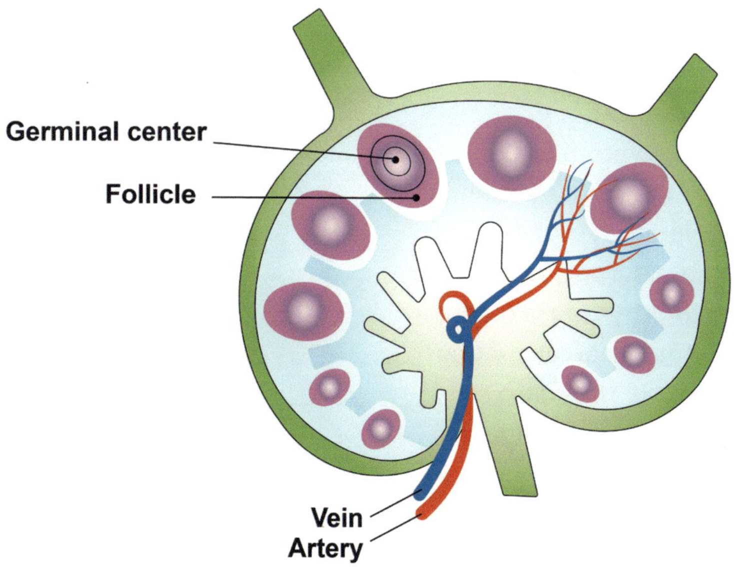

Some cancers start in immature, or still developing, cells. Follicular lymphoma starts in mature (fully developed) B cells.

How does follicular lymphoma develop?

In lymph nodes, temporary germinal centers form in response to an immune stressor, such as infection or inflammation. This is normal. But, when cells in germinal centers grow without proper regulation, they can develop into FL. In FL, excess numbers of abnormal B lymphocytes group together to form clusters (follicles) in the lymph nodes. It might be helpful to know that these short-lived germinal centers are different from those found in some subtypes of Burkitt lymphoma (BL) and diffuse large B-cell lymphoma (DLBCL).

There are 2 zones in the germinal center: light and dark.

- **B cells in the light zone are called centrocytes.** They're smaller and less in number and divide less than B cells in the dark zone.
- **B cells in the dark zone are called centroblasts.** They're larger than the cells in the light zone and reproduce (divide) more.

The types of cells found in your FL help describe its behavior.

Follicular lymphoma is a common type of non-Hodgkin lymphoma

Non-Hodgkin lymphomas start in the lymphatic system. The lymphatic, or lymph, system is part of the immune system. It includes lymph vessels, lymph nodes, tonsils, thymus, spleen, and bone marrow. Bone marrow is the main producer of blood cells.

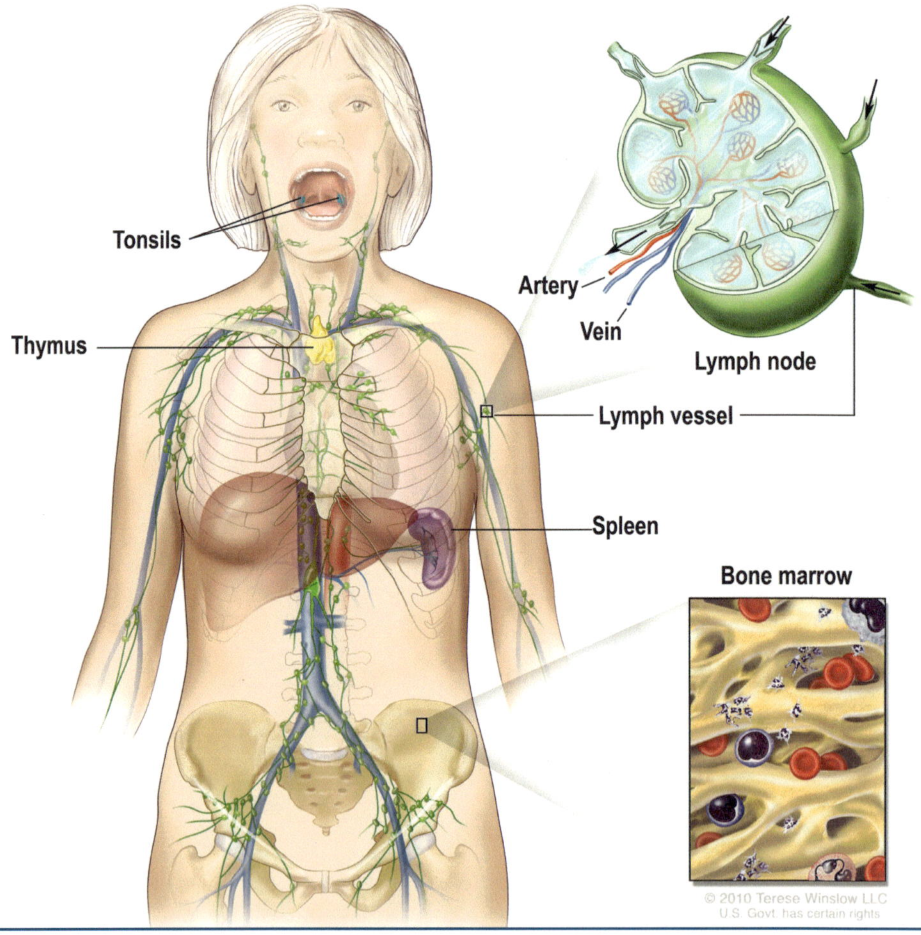

How is follicular lymphoma treated?

Since follicular lymphoma is a slow-growing (indolent) type of cancer, not everyone needs treatment right away. Often, treatment can be delayed until you have symptoms, or the lymphoma grows or changes in a way that suggests it's time to start treatment. Your care team will monitor your lymphoma for changes and suggest when it's time to begin treatment.

FL typically forms tumors in lymph nodes. However, it can form tumors in other parts of the body, such as bone marrow. This is called extranodal (outside the lymph node) disease.

Follicular lymphoma is highly treatable and may be curable in certain cases. It's treated with systemic (drug) therapy, radiation therapy, or both.

Treatment for the following types of FL are explained in this guide.

- Classic
- Uncommon (treated as classic)
- Adult pediatric type
- Transformed

How can I get the best care?

Advocate for yourself. You have an important role to play in your care. Many people feel more satisfied when they actively take part in planning their cancer care.

The NCCN Guidelines for Patients will help you play a larger role in your care. Discuss the recommendations in this guide with your care team. Ask questions about your options and share your goals and concerns.

Don't know what to ask? You're not alone. That's why we include suggested questions to ask at the end of chapters.

Keep reading to find the best care for you.

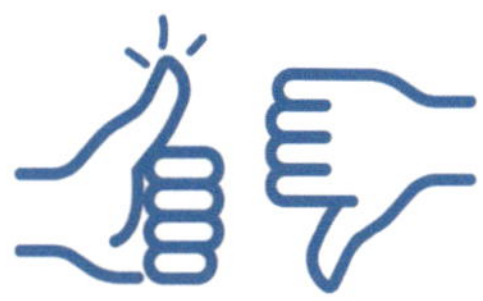

Let us know what you think!

Please take a moment to complete an online survey about the NCCN Guidelines for Patients.
NCCN.org/patients/response

2

Testing for follicular lymphoma

Accurate testing is essential to diagnose and treat follicular lymphoma (FL). This chapter presents an overview of possible tests you might receive and what to expect.

Follicular lymphoma (FL) can cause swollen lymph nodes or an enlarged spleen. Swollen lymph nodes can occur anywhere in the body, but on imaging scans they are most often found in the neck, armpit, and groin area as well as in the chest, abdomen, and pelvis. FL symptoms can include fever, night sweats, fatigue, and weight loss. These symptoms are referred to as B symptoms. Not everyone has the same symptoms. Some people don't have any symptoms.

Accurate testing is needed to diagnose and treat FL. Information on possible tests and procedures can be found in this chapter. It's okay to skip over information that doesn't interest you.

General health tests

Some general health tests are described next. For possible tests to plan treatment, see **Guide 1**.

Medical history

A medical history is a record of all health issues and treatments you've had in your life. It asks about past surgeries and current health conditions. Bring a list of old and new medicines and any over-the-counter medicines, herbals, or supplements you take. Some supplements interact with and affect medicines your care team may prescribe. Since there's often a lack of published information about how certain supplements interact with standard medicines, your care team may recommend that many of them be discontinued during treatment.

Family history

Some cancers and other diseases can run in families. Your care team will ask about the health history of family members who are blood relatives. This information is called family history. Ask members on both sides of your family about their health issues, like heart disease, cancer, and diabetes, and at what age they were diagnosed. It's important to know their specific type of cancer, where the cancer started, if it's in multiple locations, and if they had genetic testing.

Physical exam

During a physical exam, your health care provider may:

- Feel and apply pressure to parts of your body to see if organs are a normal size, are soft or hard, or cause pain when touched.
- Feel for enlarged lymph nodes in your neck, armpit, and groin.

Performance status

Performance status is a rating of a person's general level of fitness and ability to perform daily tasks. It includes whether you can walk, work, and take care of yourself. It's 1 factor taken into consideration when choosing a treatment plan.

Guide 1
Tests to diagnose follicular lymphoma and help plan treatment

Biopsy and pathology review
Immunophenotyping with immunohistochemistry and flow cytometry, and biomarker tests such as fluorescence in situ hybridization (FISH)
Physical exam with special attention to lymph node-bearing areas (including Waldeyer's ring) and to size of liver and spleen
Performance status
B symptoms (fever, drenching night sweats, and loss of more than 10 percent of body weight over 6 months)
Complete blood count with differential, lactate dehydrogenase, comprehensive metabolic panel, and hepatitis B testing
PET/CT scan (preferred) or CT with contrast of chest, abdomen, and pelvis
Pregnancy test for people of childbearing age
Possible: • Bone marrow biopsy and aspirate • Heart tests • Neck CT with contrast • Beta-2-microglobulin • Uric acid • Serum protein electrophoresis (SPEP) and other blood tests • Hepatitis C testing • Discussion of fertility preservation

Fertility (all genders)

Treatment with systemic therapy can affect your fertility, or the ability to have children. If you think you want children in the future, ask your care team how lymphoma treatment might affect your fertility.

Fertility preservation is all about keeping your options open, whether you know you want to have children later in life or aren't sure. Fertility and reproductive specialists can help you sort through what may be best for your situation.

More information on fertility preservation can be found in *NCCN Guidelines for Patients: Adolescent and Young Adult Cancer,* available at NCCN.org/patientguidelines and on the NCCN Patient Guides for Cancer app.

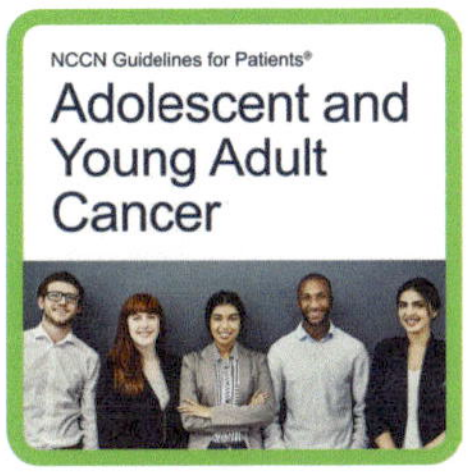

Preventing pregnancy during treatment

Preventing pregnancy during treatment is important. Lymphoma treatment can affect the ovaries, damage sperm, and hurt a developing baby. Therefore, becoming pregnant or having one's partner become pregnant during treatment should be avoided. If you're pregnant or breastfeeding at the time of your lymphoma diagnosis, treatments may need to be adjusted.

Blood tests

Blood tests check for signs of disease and how well organs are working. They require a sample of your blood, which is removed through a needle placed into your vein. Be prepared to have many blood tests during FL treatment and recovery to check treatment results, blood counts, and the health of organs like your liver and kidneys.

Some possible blood tests are described next.

It's okay to skip over information that doesn't interest you.

Complete blood count and differential

A complete blood count measures the levels of red blood cells, white blood cells, and platelets in your blood. A differential counts the number of each type of white blood cell (neutrophils, lymphocytes, monocytes, eosinophils, and basophils). It also checks if the counts are in balance with each other.

Comprehensive metabolic panel

A comprehensive metabolic panel measures different substances in your blood. It provides important information about how well your liver and kidneys are working, among other things.

Hepatitis B and hepatitis C

Hepatitis B and hepatitis C virus infections can affect the liver. A hepatitis blood test shows if you had hepatitis in the past or if you have it now. Some lymphoma treatments can wake up (or reactivate) the virus. If this happens, it can harm the liver.

Lactate dehydrogenase

Lactate dehydrogenase (LDH), or lactic acid dehydrogenase, is a protein found in most cells, including red blood cells and lung cells. Dying cells release LDH into blood. Fast-growing cells, such as lymphoma cells, also release LDH.

Pregnancy test

If planned treatment might affect pregnancy, then people who can become pregnant are given a pregnancy test before treatment begins.

SPEP

Serum protein electrophoresis (SPEP) examines specific proteins in the blood called globulins, which may be increased under certain conditions.

Uric acid

Uric acid is released by cells when DNA breaks down. It's a normal waste product that dissolves in your blood and is filtered by the kidneys where it leaves the body as urine. Too much uric acid in the body is called hyperuricemia. With FL, it can be caused by a fast turnover (cell death) of white blood cells. High uric acid might also be a side effect of treatment. Very high levels of uric acid in the blood can cause kidney stones, kidney damage, and gout (inflammation of joints).

Biopsy

A biopsy removes a tissue sample from your body for testing. It's an important part of an accurate diagnosis of lymphoma. Your sample should be reviewed by a pathologist who's an expert in the diagnosis of FL. The pathologist (or hematopathologist) will note the overall appearance and the size, shape, and type of cells and write a report. This review is often referred to as histology, histopathology, or hematopathology review. Tests are done on the biopsied cells to accurately diagnose FL.

Lymph node biopsy

A lymph node biopsy is recommended to diagnose FL. Lymph nodes can be too small to see or feel. Sometimes, lymph nodes can be swollen, enlarged, or hard or don't move when pushed (fixed or immobile). A lymph node biopsy can be done using a needle biopsy procedure or as a small surgery to remove (excise) a lymph node.

A lymph node biopsy can be done in the following ways:

- **Fine-needle aspiration** uses a very thin needle to remove a sample of tissue.
- **Core needle biopsy** uses a hollow needle to remove a larger sample of tissue.
- **Incisional biopsy** removes a small amount of tissue through a cut in the skin or body.
- **Excisional biopsy** removes the entire tumor through a cut in the skin or body.

A core needle biopsy or excisional biopsy is preferred for a follicular lymphoma diagnosis.

Bone marrow tests

Bone marrow tests might be done depending on your situation.

There are 2 types of bone marrow tests that are often done at the same time:

- Aspiration
- Biopsy

Your bone marrow is like a sponge holding liquid and cells. Aspiration takes some of the liquid and cells out of the sponge, and a biopsy removes a piece of the sponge.

Bone marrow aspiration and biopsy are bedside procedures. They aren't surgeries and don't require an operating room. Your care team will try to make you as comfortable as possible during the procedures.

The samples are usually taken from the back of the hip bone (pelvis). You'll likely lie on your belly or side. For the aspiration, a hollow needle is pushed through your skin and into the bone marrow. Liquid bone marrow is then drawn into a syringe. For the biopsy, a wider needle is used to remove a small piece of bone marrow. You may feel pain at your hip for a few days. Your skin may bruise.

Bone marrow aspiration and biopsy

Samples of bone and marrow are removed in a biopsy. A bone marrow aspiration and biopsy might be needed to learn more about your lymphoma.

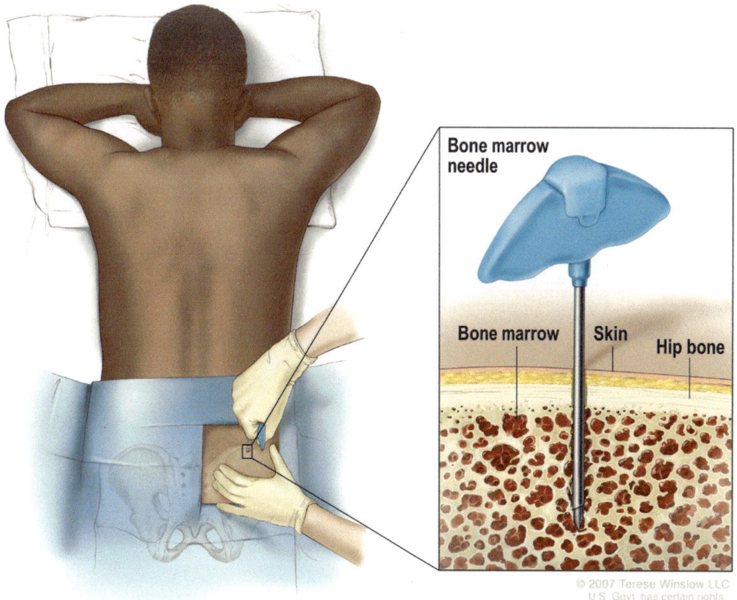

Immunophenotyping

Immunophenotyping is a process that uses antibodies to detect the presence or absence of white blood cell antigens called biomarkers. These antigens are proteins that can be found on the surface of or inside white blood cells. Certain biomarkers help identify FL or are targeted in FL treatment.

Specific groupings of antigens are normal. However, some specific patterns of antigens, called the immunophenotype, are found on abnormal cells, including FL.

Immunophenotyping can be done using specialized techniques called flow cytometry or immunohistochemistry. These techniques are used to distinguish FL from other types of lymphoma such as diffuse large B-cell lymphoma (DLBCL). The immunophenotype can change as lymphoma progresses. The FL immunophenotype is usually CD19+, CD20+, CD10+, BCL2+, CD23+/-, CD43-, CD5-, CCND1,-and BCL6+. Rare cases of FL may be CD10- or BCL2-.

Flow cytometry

Flow cytometry is a laboratory method used to detect, identify, and count specific cells. It involves adding a light-sensitive dye to cells. The dyed cells are passed through a beam of light in a machine. The machine measures the number of cells, as well as things like their size and shape.

Flow cytometry may be used on cells from circulating (peripheral) blood, bone marrow, or biopsy. The most common use of flow cytometry is to identify markers on cells, particularly in the immune system (called immunophenotyping).

Guide 2
Follicular lymphoma biomarker and genetic tests

Needed	• Biopsy and hematopathology review • IHC panel: CD20, CD3, CD5, CD10, BCL2, BCL6, CD21, or CD23 with or without cell surface marker analysis by flow cytometry: kappa/lambda, CD19, CD20, CD5, CD23, and CD10
In some cases	• Biomarker testing to detect: immunoglobulin (Ig) gene rearrangements *BCL2* rearrangements, • FISH: t(14;18), *BCL6,* 1p36, and *IRF4/MUM1* rearrangements • IHC panel: Ki-67; IRF4/MUM1 for FL grade 3, and cyclin D1 • Multigene panel including *CREBBP, EZH2, TNFRSF14,* and *STAT6* mutation

Immunohistochemistry

Immunohistochemistry (IHC) is a special staining process that involves adding a chemical marker to immune cells. The cells are then studied using a microscope. IHC looks for the immunophenotype of cells from a biopsy or tissue sample.

Biomarker tests and follicular lymphoma genetic changes

Biomarker and genetic tests are used to learn more about your type of FL, to guide treatment, and to determine the likely path your lymphoma will take (prognosis). This genetic testing is different from family history genetic testing or genetic cancer risk testing. This testing looks for changes only in the FL cells that have developed over time and not changes in the rest of your body's cells.

Inside our cells are DNA molecules. These molecules are tightly packaged into what's called a chromosome. Chromosomes contain most of the genetic information in a cell. Normal human cells contain 23 pairs of chromosomes, for a total of 46 chromosomes. Each chromosome contains thousands of genes. Most genes contain information for making a specific protein. A mutation is when something goes wrong in the genetic code. Genes are written with italics, like this: *BCL2*. Proteins are written without italics, like this: BCL2. When a gene or protein is found (expressed), it's shown with a plus sign (+), as in CD20+. When a gene or protein isn't found, it's written with a minus sign (-), as in CD20-.

FL cells sometimes have changes in genes and chromosomes that can be seen under a microscope or found with other tests.

- Testing your FL cells can gather specific information about your lymphoma to help guide treatment.
- Some results take days to weeks, but treatment may start before all results are in.

For more information on tests to diagnose FL, see **Guide 2**.

Beta-2-microglobulin tumor marker test

Beta-2-microglobulin (B2M) is a protein that can be found in the blood, urine, or fluid that surrounds your spine and brain. B2M is a type of tumor marker. Tumor markers are substances made by lymphoma cells or by normal cells in response to lymphoma in the body.

FL mutation testing

Mutation testing using methods, such as fluorescence in situ hybridization (FISH), polymerase chain reaction (PCR), and multigene panel testing (MGPT), look for changes or abnormalities that are unique to FL cells. A sample of your lymph node, blood, or bone marrow is used to see if the FL cells have any specific mutations.

Some mutations may determine the type of treatment given. Subtle, new, drug-resistant mutations may occur over time. Mutations can also happen during treatment. Some mutations lead to resistance to certain therapies. There are many possible mutations.

FISH

Fluorescence in situ hybridization (FISH) is a method that involves special dyes, called probes, that attach to pieces of DNA. Since this test doesn't need growing cells, it can be performed on bone marrow, lymph node, or a blood sample.

FISH can find translocations that are too small to be seen with other methods. A translocation occurs when parts of 2 chromosomes switch with 1 another. However, FISH can only be used for known specific changes. It can't detect all the possible changes found within the chromosomes or genes.

Translocations

Translocation is a switching of parts between 2 chromosomes. A translocation between chromosome 14 and 18 is written as t(14;18) and is found in about 9 out of 10 follicular lymphomas. It might also be referred to as *BCL2* gene rearrangement.

Gene rearrangements

Normal B cells and T cells break their DNA in certain ways to create diversity within your immune system. In a tumor, all cancer cells originate from the same cell. In FL, that cell is a B cell. Some tumors can have gene rearrangements—where part of a gene has broken off and attached to another gene, creating a new gene. For example, in a *BCL2* rearrangement, a gene from chromosome 14 moves to chromosome 18. A *BCL2* rearrangement might be written as t(14;18).

Follicular lymphoma genetic changes

Follicular lymphoma (FL) cells can have changes in genes and chromosomes. Mutation testing looks for these changes or abnormalities that are unique to FL cells. Examples of such changes are called deletion, insertion, amplification, translocation (rearrangement), and point mutation. Most follicular lymphomas test positive for t(14;18) or *BCL2.*

- ✓ **Amplification** – When a part or whole chromosome or gene is increased (for example, duplicated)
- ✓ **Deletion** – When part of a chromosome or gene is missing
- ✓ **Insertion** – When a new part of a chromosome or gene is included
- ✓ **Inversion** – When parts within 1 chromosome are switched
- ✓ **Point mutation** – When part of a gene is changed
- ✓ **Chromosome translocation and gene rearrangement** – When parts between 2 chromosomes are switched. When described at the chromosome level, it's called a translocation. When described at the gene level, it's called rearrangement. For example, the chromosome translocation is written as t(14;18) and its gene rearrangement is written as *IGH::BCL2.*

Imaging tests

Imaging tests take pictures of the inside of your body to look for cancer, enlarged lymph nodes, or other abnormalities that might suggest lymphoma. A radiologist, an expert in interpreting imaging tests, will write a report for your care team.

Possible imaging tests are described next. They're listed in alphabetical order and not in order of importance. You won't have all of these tests.

Contrast material

Contrast material is a substance used to improve the quality of CT and MRI imaging scans. It's used to make the pictures clearer. Not all imaging tests require contrast, but many do.

Contrast might be taken by mouth (oral) or given through a vein (intravenously, or IV).The types of contrast vary and are different for CT and MRI.

Tell your care team if you've had allergic reactions to contrast in the past. This is important. You might be given medicines to avoid the effects of those allergies. Contrast might not be used if you have a serious allergy or if your kidneys aren't working well.

CT scan

A CT, or CAT, scan uses x-rays and computer technology to take pictures of the inside of the body. It takes many x-rays of the same body part from different angles. All the images are combined to make 1 detailed picture. A CT scan of your chest, abdomen, and pelvis may be one of the tests to look for lymphoma. In most cases, contrast is used.

MRI scan

An MRI scan uses radio waves and powerful magnets to take pictures of the inside of the body. MRI doesn't use radiation. Because of the very strong magnets used in the MRI machine, tell the technologist if you have any metal or a pacemaker in your body. Contrast is often used.

MRI scans take longer than CT scans. A closed MRI has a capsule-like design where the magnet surrounds you. An open MRI has a magnetic top and bottom, which allows for an opening on each end. Closed MRIs are more common than open MRIs, so if you have claustrophobia (a fear of enclosed spaces), be sure to talk to your care team.

An MRI may be used to evaluate the brain and the spinal cord.

PET scan

A PET scan uses a radioactive substance called a tracer. A tracer is injected into a vein to see where lymphoma cells are in the body and how much sugar they take up, since malignant cells metabolize sugar faster than normal cells. This gives an idea about how fast these cells are growing. Lymphoma shows up as bright spots on PET scans. However, not all tumors appear on a PET scan. Also, not all bright spots are lymphoma. It's normal for the brain, heart, kidneys, and bladder to be bright on PET. Inflammation or infection can also show up as a bright spot. When a PET scan is combined with CT, it's called a PET/CT scan.

Heart tests

Heart, or cardiac, tests are used to see how well the heart works. These tests might be used to monitor treatment side effects or to measure your heart function before you start treatment. You might be referred to a heart specialist called a cardiologist.

Key points

- Be prepared to have many blood tests during follicular lymphoma (FL) treatment and recovery to check blood counts, treatment results, and the health of your organs.
- A biopsy removes a sample of tissue for testing. It's an important part of an accurate FL diagnosis.
- A sample from your biopsy may undergo lab tests to learn more about your FL and choose the best treatment for you.
- Immunophenotyping is used to distinguish FL from other types of lymphoma.
- Biomarker and genetic tests are used to learn more about your type of FL, to guide treatment, and to determine the likely path your lymphoma will take (prognosis).
- Almost everyone with FL has a t(14:18) chromosome translocation or excess levels of the BCL2 protein (BCL2+) in their tumor. A chromosome translocation is the switching of pieces of 2 chromosomes within the lymphoma cells.
- Certain treatments can affect heart function. Heart tests might be used to see how well your heart works.

Questions to ask

- What can you tell me about my type of follicular lymphoma?
- Is there a cancer center or hospital nearby that specializes in treating lymphoma?
- What type of biopsy will I have?
- What types of biomarker and genetic tests will be done on the biopsy sample?
- When will the test results be ready and who will discuss them with me?

What's next?

The next chapter provides information on the types of treatment and what to expect from treatment.

How this guide can help you

Making decisions about cancer care is stressful. There's a lot to learn, and you don't know what the future holds.

Use this guide to get the information and support you need.

Patients, doctors, and other health care professionals trust the NCCN Guidelines for Patients. This guide uses clear, everyday language to explain current cancer care recommendations made by respected experts in the field. Their recommendations are based on the latest research and practices at leading cancer centers.

Your health is unique to you, so your cancer care should be, too. As you read this guide, you'll learn which treatments are likely to provide the best results for you. And you'll be better prepared to talk with your care team

3

Types of treatment

There's more than one treatment for follicular lymphoma (FL). This chapter presents an overview of the possible types of treatment and what to expect. Not everyone will receive the same treatment. Treatment options are based on many factors.

Your care team

Treating lymphoma takes a team approach. Treatment decisions should involve a team of health care and psychosocial care professionals from different backgrounds who have knowledge and experience in your type of lymphoma. This team is united in planning and implementing your treatment.

Types of follicular lymphoma

Treatment for the following types of follicular lymphoma (FL) are described in this guide.

Classic FL

Classic follicular lymphoma (cFL) is grade 1, 2, 3A, or 3B. Grade 3B is usually treated as diffuse large B-cell lymphoma (DLBCL). Grade is further explained on page 23. Almost everyone with FL has a t(14;18) chromosome translocation or excess levels of the BCL2 protein (BCL2+) in their tumor. A chromosome translocation is the switching of part of 1 chromosome with another chromosome within the lymphoma cells. Treatment for cFL can be found in *Chapter 5: Classic follicular lymphoma*.

"At first I was overwhelmed by my diagnosis, as I think we all are. But I found a specialist, and as I learned more about FL treatment, my life remained relatively stable."

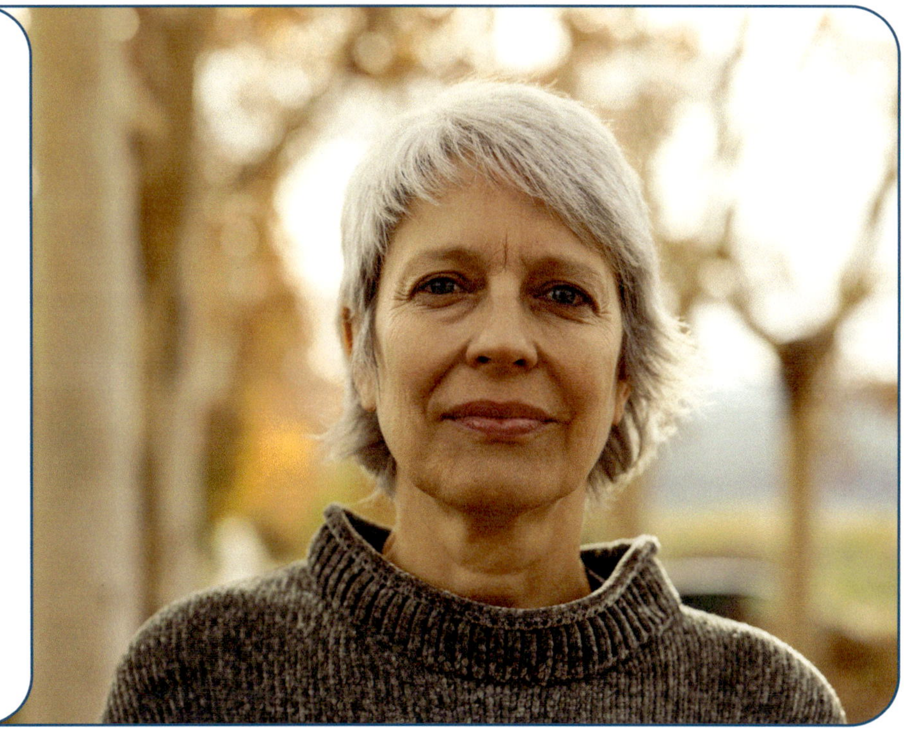

Uncommon FL

When FL has uncommon disease features or is t(14;18)-negative, it might be called uncommon FL (uFL). It's treated as classic FL as found in *Chapter 5: Classic follicular lymphoma*.

Pediatric-type FL

Pediatric-type FL (PTFL) usually occurs in children but can also occur in adults. Usually, only 1 lymph node is enlarged in the head and neck region, and there might be no symptoms. Specific treatment for PTFL can be found in *Chapter 6: Adult pediatric-type follicular lymphoma*.

Transformed FL

FL can transform into a more aggressive lymphoma called diffuse large B-cell lymphoma (DLBCL). This means your slow-growing FL has turned into a large-celled, fast-growing lymphoma. Transformed FL can occur before, during, or after treatment. In DLBCL, tumors are commonly found in lymph nodes, spleen, liver, bone marrow, or other tissues and organs. Treatment for transformed FL can be found in *Chapter 7: Transformed follicular lymphoma*.

Treatment overview

Follicular lymphoma (FL) is highly treatable and may be curable in certain circumstances. Often, treatment for FL can wait until you have symptoms. However, most people with FL don't have symptoms when starting treatment. This is because they might not have symptoms even though the lymphoma has grown or progressed (called progressive lymphadenopathy).

Treatment for FL usually consists of systemic therapy, radiation therapy, or both. Systemic therapy is drug therapy that works throughout the body. Some types include chemotherapy, targeted therapy, and immunotherapy. Radiation therapy is delivered to specific parts of the body, depending on where FL is found.

The choice of therapy takes into consideration many factors, including age, other serious health issues, expected effectiveness and side effects, and future treatment possibilities like CAR T-cell therapy or hematopoietic cell transplant (HCT). Your care team will examine all the information about your condition to come up with a proposed treatment regimen that's best for you. You're an important and critical member of your treatment team and your preferences about treatment are also very important.

Every lymphoma treatment has well-known side effects. Before you make any treatment decisions, your doctor will explain in detail the potential benefits and side effects of a treatment regimen. During and after treatment, you'll be closely monitored for signs and symptoms of lymphoma and side effects of treatment, including long-term side effects. Tell you care team about any new or worsening symptoms.

Observation without treatment

Some slow-growing (indolent) lymphomas like FL don't require immediate treatment. During observation, your care team will monitor for changes in your health or signs that your lymphoma has grown or progressed. Observation is sometimes called active surveillance or watch and wait.

Remission

The goal of treatment is remission. There are different types of remission. When no signs of lymphoma can be seen on imaging tests or with a bone marrow biopsy, it's called a complete response or complete remission. Remission can be short-term (temporary) or long-lasting (permanent). In a partial response, lymphoma is still present but it's reduced in size.

Follicular lymphoma can go through long periods of remission followed by relapses. FL can also regress, or get smaller, on its own without treatment. This isn't completely understood, but it's not uncommon for FL to fluctuate in size.

Relapse

When FL returns after a period of remission, it's called a relapse. The goal of treatment is to achieve remission again. Depending on the pace of tumor growth and the location and size of the tumor, you might not need treatment right away.

FL might relapse more than once. A relapse may or may not be serious. It's important to ask about your prognosis.

Refractory

When FL remains and doesn't respond to treatment, it's called refractory or resistant cancer. This lymphoma may be resistant at the start of treatment, or it may become resistant during treatment. Refractory disease is very serious. It's important to ask about your prognosis.

Surveillance and monitoring

You'll be monitored during and after treatment. Surveillance watches for any changes in your condition. You'll have tests during surveillance to check for relapse. You might hear it called active surveillance or observation.

Treatment planning

This section explains scoring systems used to plan FL treatment. It's important to have regular talks with your care team about your goals for treatment and your treatment plan.

Grades

The types of cells found in your FL help determine the grade. The grades of FL are 1, 2, 3A, and 3B. The more centroblasts, the higher the grade. Grades 1, 2, and 3A contain mixtures of centrocytes (small cells) and centroblasts (large cells), whereas grade 3B contains only centroblasts.

There are 2 systems used to grade FL: 2022 World Health Organization classification (WHO5) and International Consensus Classification (ICC). In WHO5, grades 1, 2, and 3A are called classic FL. The ICC calls grades 1 and 2 classic FL..

In this guide:

- FL grade 1 and 2 are treated as classic FL. Treatment for classic FL is found in Chapter 5.
- FL grade 3A might be treated as classic FL or DLBCL.
- FL grade 3B is now called follicular high-grade B-cell lymphoma and is treated as DLBCL.

Treatment for DLBCL can be found in the *NCCN Guidelines for Patients: Diffuse Large B-Cell Lymphomas*, available at NCCN.org/patientguidelines and on the NCCN Patient Guides for Cancer app.

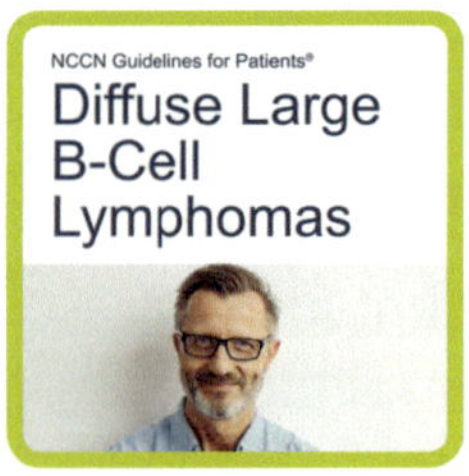

Stages

Cancer staging is used to reflect prognosis and help guide treatment decisions. Prognosis is the likely course your lymphoma will take. In follicular lymphoma (FL), your age, the number and location of lymph nodes affected by cancer, blood test results, and other factors play a role in prognosis. In addition, treatment decisions are based on histology and the results of FL biomarker and genetic tests. Histology is the overall appearance and size, shape, and type of cells.

There are different kinds of staging systems. The Lugano Modification of Ann Arbor Staging System is used for FL.

In general, stages are as follows:

- **Stage 1** – Disease found in 1 lymph node or a group of nearby lymph nodes.
- **Stage 2** – Disease found in 2 or more lymph node groups on the same side of the diaphragm.
- **Stage 3** – Disease found in lymph nodes above and below the diaphragm on the same side of the body, or disease found in nodes above the diaphragm and in the spleen.
- **Stage 4** – Disease that has spread outside the lymphatic system to other parts of the body.

International Prognostic Index

The International Prognostic Index (IPI) is a scoring system for prognosis in people with lymphoma. A prognosis is the likely course your disease will take. A follicular lymphoma IPI (FLIPI-1) is based on age, Ann Arbor cancer stage, hemoglobin and lactate dehydrogenase results, and the number of lymph node sites with lymphoma.

GELF criteria

The Groupe d'Etude des Lymphomes Folliculaires (GELF) criteria measure tumor burden, or the amount of lymphoma in the body. It helps your care team decide if treatment should start right way.

According to GELF criteria, there's high tumor burden if you have any of the following:

- Cancer 3 centimeters (cm) or larger in 3 or more lymph node areas
- A tumor mass 7 cm or larger (bulky disease) found anywhere in the body

- B symptoms (such as fever, night sweats, fatigue, and weight loss)
- Enlarged spleen (splenomegaly)
- Fluid build-up around the lungs (pleural effusion) or in the abdomen (peritoneal ascites)
- Low white blood cell (leukopenia) and/or platelet (thrombocytopenia) counts
- Leukemia

Chemotherapy

Chemotherapy kills fast-dividing cells throughout the body, including lymphoma cells and some normal cells. More than 1 chemotherapy may be used to treat FL. When only 1 drug is used, it's called a single-agent regimen. When 2 or more drugs are used, it's called a combination or multi-agent regimen.

Some chemotherapy drugs are liquids given through a vein or injected under the skin with a needle. Other chemotherapy drugs are given as a pill. The dose differs between people because it's based on body weight and height.

Most chemotherapy is given in cycles of days of treatment followed by days of rest. This allows the body to recover before the next cycle. Cycles vary in length depending on which drugs are used. The number of treatment days per cycle and the total number of cycles also vary. You might spend time in the hospital during treatment.

About NCCN recomendations for therapy

Follicular lymphoma is treated with systemic therapy, radiation therapy, or both.

All treatments listed in this guide are deemed recommended and appropriate, by our NCCN panel members for follicular lymphoma. This panel often assign levels of preferrence to the treatment recommendations as described below.

- **Preferred therapies** have the most evidence they may work better and be safer than other therapies.
- **Other recommended therapies** can provide effective results but may have less evidence, more side effects, or may not work quite as well as preferred therapies.
- **Therapies used in certain cases** work best for individuals with specific cancer features or health circumstances.

Immunotherapy

Immunotherapy increases the activity of your immune system. By doing so, it improves your body's ability to find and destroy lymphoma cells. Immunotherapy can be given alone or with other types of treatment.

Antibody therapy

Monoclonal antibody therapy and bispecific antibody therapy use antibodies to help the body fight lymphoma, infection, or other diseases. Antibodies are proteins made by the immune system that bind to specific markers (proteins) on cells or tissues.

Monoclonal antibody therapy

A monoclonal antibody (mAb) is made from a unique white blood cell, such as B cell or T cell. mAbs used in FL treatment may kill lymphoma cells directly or help the immune system kill lymphoma cells.

CD19-targeting monoclonal antibody therapy

Tafasitamab-cxix (Monjuvi) is used to treat transformed FL or high-grade B-cell lymphomas by targeting the CD19 protein.

CD20-targeting monoclonal antibody therapy

CD20-targeting mAbs (also called anti-CD20 mAbs), such as rituximab (Rituxan) and obinutuzumab (Gazyva), work against the protein CD20 found on the surface of B cells. The drug binds to the CD20 protein, causing cell death.

Warnings about supplements and drug interactions

Some supplements and foods can affect the ability of a drug used to treat follicular lymphoma to do its job. This is called a drug interaction. Since there's often a lack of published information about how certain supplements interact with standard medicines, your care team may recommend that many of them be discontinued during treatment

Also, certain medicines can affect the ability of a drug to do its job. Antacids, heart or blood pressure medicine, and antidepressants are just some of the medicines that might interact with systemic therapy or supportive care medicines given during systemic drug therapy.

Therefore, it's very important to tell your care team about all medicines, vitamins, over-the-counter drugs, herbals, or supplements you're taking.

Bring a list with you to every visit.

Bispecific antibody therapy

Bispecific antibodies bind to 2 different proteins (CD20 and CD3 antigen) at the same time—one on the immune T cells and the other on the lymphoma cells. Bispecific antibody therapy treats lymphoma by engaging and activating T cells and redirecting them to the lymphoma site. Bispecific examples include epcoritamab-bysp (Epkinly), mosunetuzumab-axgb (Lunsumio), and glofitamab-gxbm (Columvi).

CD19-targeting CAR T-cell immunotherapy

CAR T-cell therapy is a personalized form of immunotherapy called cellular therapy. T cells from your body are removed, and then they're trained to fight the lymphoma by adding a CAR (chimeric antigen receptor) to the T cells. This programs the T cells to find lymphoma cells. The programmed T cells are infused back into your body after a brief course of chemotherapy (called lymphodepleting chemotherapy). Chemotherapy is needed too get the body ready to accept the CAR T-cells. This treatment isn't for everyone.

CAR T-cell therapy is one way to target the CD19 protein found on almost all B-cell lymphomas, including FL. CD19-targeting CAR T-cell therapy options for FL include axicabtagene ciloleucel (Yescarta), lisocabtagene maraleucel (Breyanzi), and tisagenlecleucel (Kymriah).

For information on CAR T-cell therapy side effects, see *NCCN Guidelines for Patients: Immunotherapy Side Effects*, available at NCCN.org/patientguidelines and on the NCCN Patient Guides for Cancer app.

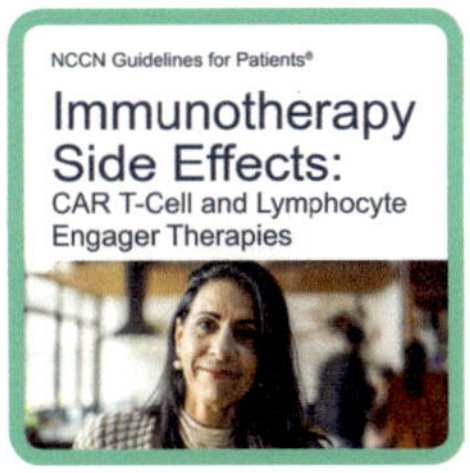

Chemoimmunotherapy

Chemoimmunotherapy, also called immunochemotherapy, combines chemotherapy and immunotherapy drugs to treat cancer. There are several chemoimmunotherapy regimens used to treat FL.

Examples include:

- Bendamustine plus obinutuzumab or rituximab
- CHOP (cyclophosphamide, doxorubicin, vincristine, and prednisone) plus obinutuzumab or rituximab
- CVP (cyclophosphamide, vincristine, and prednisone) plus obinutuzumab or rituximab

Targeted therapy

Targeted therapy focuses on specific or unique features of lymphoma cells. Targeted therapies seek out how lymphoma cells grow, divide, and move in the body. These drugs stop or inhibit the action of molecules that help lymphoma cells grow and/or survive.

Other systemic therapies

Antibody-drug conjugate

An antibody-drug conjugate (ADC) delivers cell-specific chemotherapy. It attaches to a protein found on the outside of the lymphoma cell, then enters the cell. Once inside the cell, chemotherapy is released. Loncastuximab tesirine-lpyl (Zynlonta) is an ADC that targets the CD19 protein. Polatuzumab vedotin-piiq (Polivy) targets the CD79b protein. An ADC might be used for transformed FL.

Immune modulator

An immune modulator changes your immune system so it can work more effectively, especially when combined with monoclonal antibodies. Lenalidomide (Revlimid) is an example of an immune modulator that's used commonly with rituximab, obinutuzumab, epcoritamab-bysp, or tafasitamab.

Standard of care is the best-known way to treat a particular disease based on past clinical trials. There may be more than one treatment regimen that is considered standard of care. Ask your care team what treatment options are available and if a clinical trial might be right for you.

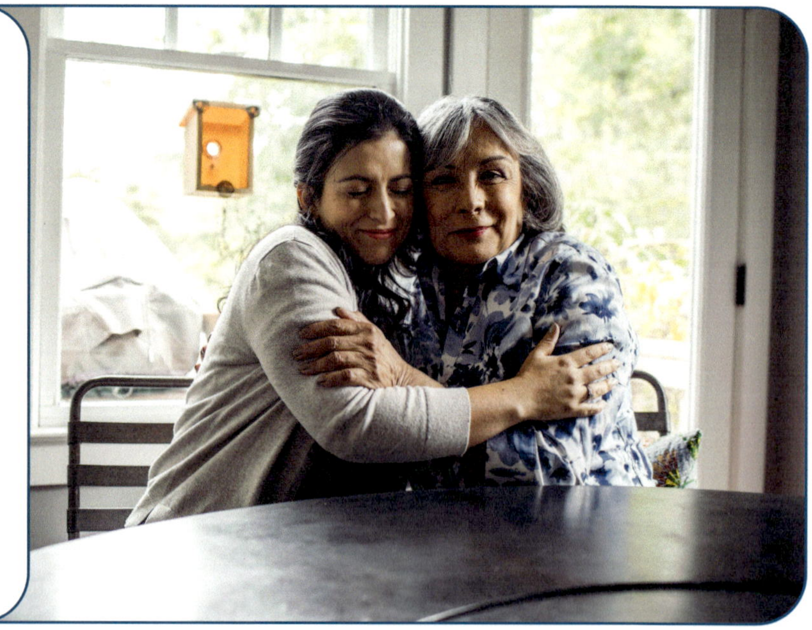

Radiation therapy

Radiation therapy (RT) uses high energy to kill lymphoma cells and shrink tumors. RT may be used to cure lymphoma (curative treatment), or as supportive care or palliative care (palliative treatment) to help ease the pain or discomfort caused by lymphoma. The dose of radiation typically prescribed for follicular lymphoma is very low.

Most FLs are very sensitive to radiation. Because of this, radiation therapy is widely used to treat FL, especially as a curative treatment for early-stage disease, or for palliative treatment at any stage.

The first step of RT is simulation (or mapping), a dedicated CT scan done at the radiation oncology department. Your radiation oncologist uses that scan and computer software to create a 3D radiation treatment plan. During treatment, radiation in the form of beams shaped to the tumor area is delivered from outside the body by a device.

Depending on your situation, you may receive as little as 1 treatment or as many as 20 or more. Treatment is given in small daily doses, typically Monday through Friday. Some people receive 2 treatments a day.

- **Involved-site radiation therapy**, a technique that treats the area surrounding the tumor, is currently the typical approach to FL treatment.

You'll see your radiation oncologist at least once a week during RT. During these visits, the doctor will examine you and ask how you're feeling.

Most follicular lymphomas are very sensitive to radiation therapy

Radiation therapy is widely used to treat follicular lymphoma, especially as a curative treatment for early-stage disease, or for palliative treatment at any stage.

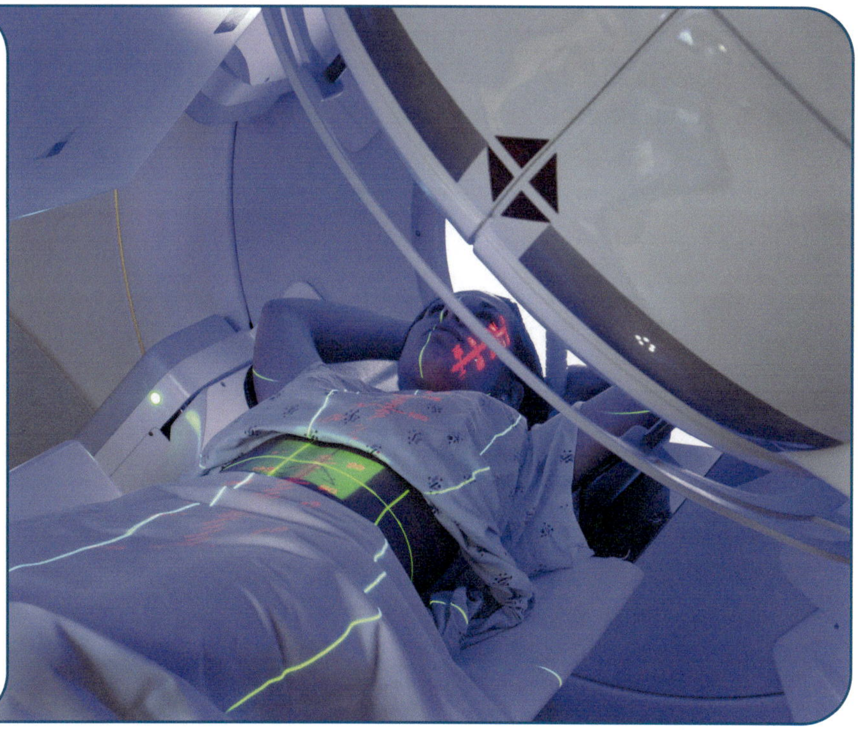

Hematopoietic cell transplant

A hematopoietic cell transplant (HCT), or stem cell transplant, is a cellular therapy that replaces a person's bone marrow and immune system with donor cells. More specifically, an HCT replaces hematopoietic stem cells that have been destroyed by high doses of chemotherapy and/or radiation therapy as part of the transplant process. A hematopoietic stem cell is an immature cell that can develop into any type of blood cell. HCTs are performed in specialized centers.

- HCTs are only given in very specific cases for follicular lymphoma. Ask your care team why.

There are 2 types of HCTs:

- **Autologous** – Stem cells come from you. It's called high-dose therapy with autologous stem cell rescue (HDT/ASCR).
- **Allogeneic** – Stem cells come from a donor who may or may not be related to you. Compared to an autologous HCT, an allogeneic HCT introduces new immune cells from a donor, which may be able to detect and eliminate lymphoma cells better than your immune system. An allogeneic HCT is preferred over an autologous HCT in FL.

Both types of HCTs can be part of the treatment of FL, but their use has waned over the past few years because of the development of new cellular therapies, such as CAR T-cell therapy and bispecific antibody therapy. However, these transplants can still be curative options if the other treatments weren't successful and may be preferred in certain people.

Allogeneic HCT

An allogeneic HCT uses healthy stem cells from a donor. Before HCT, treatment is needed to destroy bone marrow cells. This is called conditioning, and it creates room for the transplanted healthy stem cells. It also weakens the immune system, so your body won't kill the transplanted cells. Chemotherapy is used for conditioning. Radiation therapy may also be given as part of conditioning treatment.

After conditioning, you'll receive a transfusion of the healthy stem cells from a donor who's matched to you. A transfusion is a slow injection of blood products into a vein. This can take several hours. The transplanted stem cells travel to your bone marrow and grow. New, healthy blood cells form. This is called engraftment. It usually takes about 2 to 4 weeks. Until then, you'll have little or no immune defense. You may need to stay in a very clean room at the hospital or be given antibiotics to prevent or treat infection. Transfusions are also possible. A red blood cell transfusion is used to prevent bleeding and to treat anemia (below normal red blood cell count). A platelet transfusion is used to treat a low platelet count or bleeding. While waiting for the cells to engraft, you'll likely feel tired and weak. This treatment has very serious and life-threatening side effects.

The goal of the transplant is for the new immune system to recognize the lymphoma as foreign and destroy it and to provide you with a new, healthy immune system.

Clinical trials

You may also be able to receive treatment through a clinical trial. A clinical trial is a type of medical research study. After being developed and tested in a lab, potential new ways of treating cancer need to be studied in people.

If found to be safe and effective in a clinical trial, a drug, device, or treatment approach may be approved by the U.S. FDA.

Everyone with cancer should carefully consider all of the treatment options available for their cancer type, including standard treatments and clinical trials. Talk to your doctor about whether a clinical trial may make sense for you.

Phases

Most cancer clinical trials focus on treatment and are done in phases.

- **Phase 1** trials study the safety and side effects of an investigational drug or treatment approach.
- **Phase 2** trials study how well the drug or approach works against a specific type of cancer.
- **Phase 3** trials test the drug or approach against a standard treatment. If the results are good, it may be approved by the FDA.
- **Phase 4** trials study the safety and benefit of an FDA-approved treatment.

Finding a clinical trial

In the United States

NCCN Cancer Centers
NCCN.org/cancercenters

The National Cancer Institute (NCI)
cancer.gov/about-cancer/treatment/clinical-trials/search

Worldwide

The U.S. National Library of Medicine (NLM)
clinicaltrials.gov

Need help finding a clinical trial?

NCI's Cancer Information Service (CIS)
1.800.4.CANCER (1.800.422.6237)
cancer.gov/contact

Who can enroll?

It depends on the clinical trial's rules, called eligibility criteria. The rules may be about age, cancer type and stage, treatment history, or general health. They ensure that participants are alike in specific ways and that the trial is as safe as possible for the participants.

Informed consent

Clinical trials are managed by a research team. This group of experts will review the study with you in detail, including its purpose and the risks and benefits of joining. All of this information is also provided in an informed consent form. Read the form carefully and ask questions before signing it. Take time to discuss it with people you trust. Keep in mind that you can leave and seek treatment outside of the clinical trial at any time.

Will I get a placebo?

Placebos (inactive versions of real medicines) are almost never used alone in lymphoma clinical trials. It's common to receive either a placebo added to a standard treatment, or a new drug with a standard treatment.

Are clinical trials free?

There's no fee to enroll in a clinical trial. The study sponsor pays for research-related costs, including the study drug. But you may need to pay for other services, like transportation or childcare, due to extra appointments. Most clinical trials do not cover routine CT scans or other imaging tests. Unless they were being done specifically for the trial. During the trial, you'll continue to receive standard cancer care. This care is usually covered by insurance.

Key points

- Follicular lymphoma (FL) is highly treatable and may be curable in certain circumstances. Often, treatment for FL can wait until you have symptoms. However, most people with FL don't have symptoms when starting treatment.
- FL can regress, or get smaller, on its own without treatment. This isn't completely understood, but it's common for FL to fluctuate in size.
- Treatment for FL usually consists of systemic therapy, radiation therapy, or both. The goal of treatment is to achieve a complete response or remission.
- Systemic therapy works throughout the body. It includes chemotherapy, targeted therapy, and immunotherapy.
- Radiation therapy uses high energy to kill lymphoma cells and shrink tumors.
- A clinical trial is a type of research that studies a treatment to see how safe it is and how well it works.

Questions to ask

- What type of follicular lymphoma do I have, and what can you tell me about the grade, stage, and other features?
- What experience do you have treating follicular lymphoma?
- How long will treatment take, and in what order will it be given?
- What websites about my condition do you recommend? Is there any information I can take home to read?
- Are there resources to help me pay for treatment or other care I may need?

What's next?

Now that you've read about the different types of treatment and what to expect, the next chapter talks about some general side effects of treatment and what might be done to manage those effects.

"You'll get through this! Bring someone with you to every appointment: they can help take notes and keep a list of your questions to ensure they're answered. More importantly, they'll be there to provide comfort for you during this difficult time."

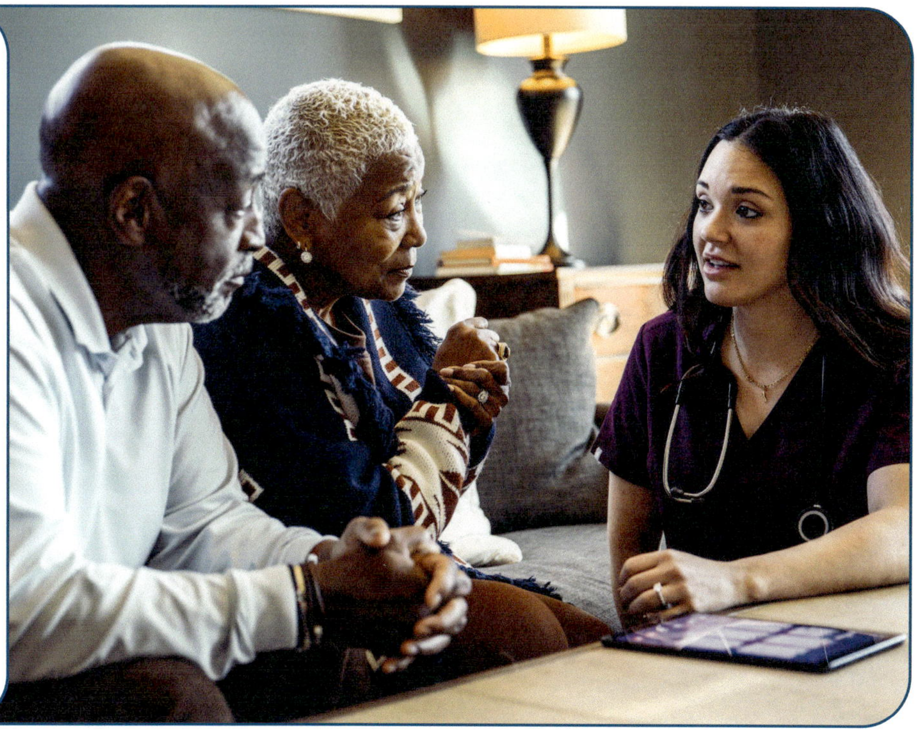

4
Supportive care

Supportive care helps manage the symptoms of follicular lymphoma and the side effects of treatment. This chapter discusses supportive care for possible treatment side effects.

What is supportive care?

Supportive care is an important part of cancer care. The goal is to improve your quality of life during and after cancer treatment. Supportive care is for everyone with cancer and their families, not just for those at the end of life.

Supportive care includes a wide range of services. Supportive care prevents or manages the symptoms of cancer and the side effects of cancer treatment, like pain and cancer-related fatigue. It also addresses the mental, social, emotional, and spiritual concerns faced by people with cancer.

Supportive care provides help with additional needs, such as:

- Making treatment decisions
- Coordinating your care
- Paying for care
- Planning for advanced care and end of life

Some health care professionals refer to palliative care as supportive care. They think these types of care are alike or overlap. Others think there are important differences, but both help people with cancer to live as well as they can. Your cancer center may have palliative care specialists, who can give you additional support and help coordinate your supportive care needs.

Supportive care resources

More information on supportive care is available at NCCN.org/patientguidelines and on the NCCN Patient Guides for Cancer app.

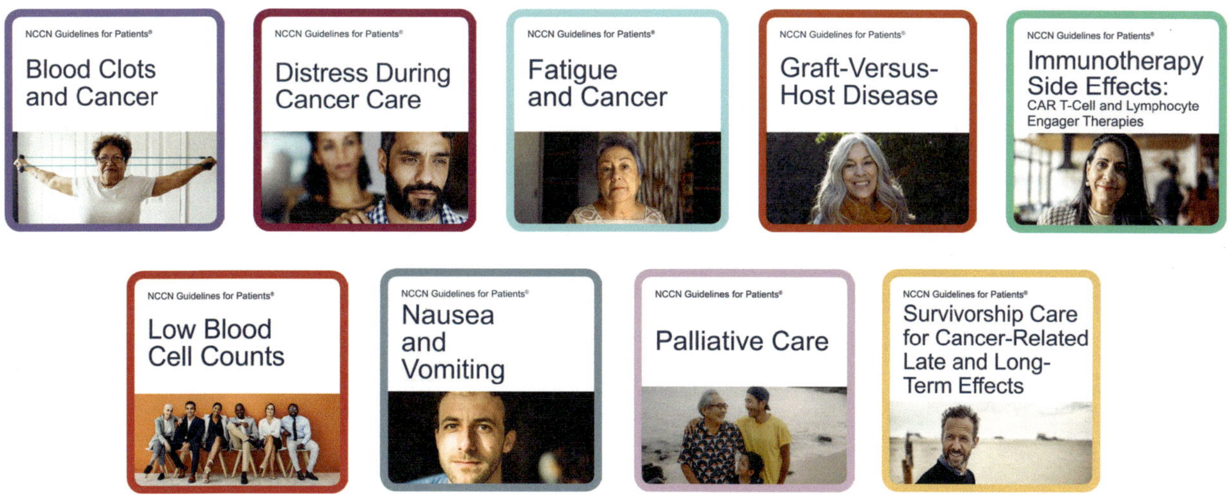

Read more about the types of support you may receive in *NCCN Guidelines for Patients: Palliative Care*, available at NCCN.org/patientguidelines and on the NCCN Patient Guides for Cancer app.

Tell your care team about any new or worsening symptoms so they can be managed.

Side effects

All lymphoma treatments can cause unwanted health issues called side effects. Side effects depend on many factors. These factors include the drug type and dose, length of treatment, and the person. Some side effects are very serious. Tell your care team about any new or worsening symptoms.

Some common side effects are described next.

Blood clots

Cancer can cause blood clots to form. This can block blood flow and oxygen delivery to parts of the body. Blood clots can break loose and travel to other parts of the body, causing breathing problems, stroke, or other health issues.

Cytokine release syndrome

Cytokine release syndrome only happens during treatment with CAR T-cell therapy or bispecific antibody therapy. It's caused by a large, rapid release of cytokines from immune cells. Cytokines are proteins made and released by the body as a response to infection, inflammation, or some treatments. Signs and symptoms include fever, muscle aches, nausea, headache, rash, fast heartbeat, low blood pressure, and trouble breathing.

Diarrhea

Diarrhea, frequent and watery bowel movements, is a common side effect. Your care team will tell you how to manage diarrhea. When it occurs, it's important to drink lots of fluids.

Emotional distress

Depression, anxiety, and sleeping issues are common during a lymphoma diagnosis. Talk to your care team and those with whom you feel most comfortable about how you're feeling. There are services, people, and medicine that may be recommended to help relieve your distress.

Fatigue

Fatigue is a state of physical or mental tiredness that can feel like a lack of energy, motivation, or stamina. Fatigue may be caused by lymphoma, or it may be a side effect of treatment. Let your care team know how you're feeling and if fatigue is getting in the way of doing the things you enjoy. Eating a balanced diet, exercise, yoga, acupuncture, and massage therapy can help. You might be referred to a nutritionist or dietitian to help with fatigue. It's important to try to stay active.

GVHD

Graft-versus-host disease (GVHD) is a possible side effect of a hematopoietic cell transplant (HCT). In GVHD, the donor cells attack your normal, healthy tissue, such as your organs and skin. There are treatments for GVHD.

Hair loss

Chemotherapy may cause hair loss (alopecia) all over your body—not just on your scalp. Some chemotherapy drugs are more likely than others to cause hair loss. Dosage might also affect the amount of hair loss. Most of the time, hair loss from chemotherapy is temporary. Hair often regrows 3 to 6 months after treatment ends. Your hair may be a different shade or texture at first. Scalp cooling (or scalp hypothermia) might help lessen hair loss in people receiving certain types of chemotherapy.

Hand-foot syndrome

Hand-foot syndrome is a common side effect of chemotherapy. Small amounts of chemotherapy leak out of very small blood vessels called capillaries in the palms of the hands and soles of the feet. It causes redness, swelling, and pain. Sometimes blisters appear. You'll want to protect your hands and feet by applying moisturizer or lotion.

Hypersensitivity, allergy, and anaphylaxis

Hypersensitivity is an exaggerated response by the immune system to a drug or other substance. This can include hives, skin welts, and trouble breathing. An allergy is an immune reaction to a substance that normally is harmless or would not cause an immune response in most people. An allergic response may cause symptoms, such as itching or inflammation (swelling). Anaphylaxis or anaphylactic shock is a severe and possible life-threatening allergic reaction.

Infections

Infections are more common and more severe in people with a weakened immune system. Drug treatment for follicular lymphoma can reduce the body's natural defense against infections. If not treated early, infections can be fatal.

Neutropenia, a low number of white blood cells that often occurs during treatment, can lead to frequent or severe infections. When someone with neutropenia develops a fever, it's called febrile neutropenia (FN). A fever is a temperature of over 100.4° F. With FN, your risk of infection may be higher than normal. This is because a low number of white blood cells leads to a reduced ability to fight infections. Sometimes the infection can be from bacteria entering the bloodstream, which is very dangerous. FN is a side effect of some types of systemic therapy. Ask your care team how to prevent FN, what to look for, and what to do in an emergency.

Loss of appetite

The side effects from lymphoma treatment and the stress of having FL might cause you to feel not hungry or sick to your stomach (nauseated). You might have a sore mouth or difficulty swallowing.

Healthy eating is important during treatment. It includes eating a balanced diet, eating the right amount of food, and drinking enough fluids. A registered dietitian who's an expert in nutrition and food can help.

Low blood cell counts

Some lymphoma treatments can cause low blood cell counts.

- **Anemia** is a condition where your body doesn't have enough healthy red blood cells, resulting in less oxygen being carried to your organs. You might tire easily if you're anemic.
- **Neutropenia** is a decrease in neutrophils, a type of white blood cell. This puts you at risk of infection.
- **Thrombocytopenia** is a condition where there aren't enough platelets found in the blood. This puts you at risk of bleeding.

Lymphedema

Lymphedema is a condition in which lymph fluid builds up in tissues and causes swelling. It may be caused when part of the lymph system is damaged or blocked. Lymphomas that block lymph vessels can also cause lymphedema. Swelling usually develops slowly over time. If you have lymphedema, you may be referred to an expert in lymphedema management. The swelling may be reduced by exercise, massage, compression devices, and other means.

Nausea and vomiting

Nausea and vomiting are common side effects of treatment. You may be given medicine to prevent nausea and vomiting.

Neuropathy and neurotoxicity

Some treatments can damage the nervous system (neurotoxicity), causing neuropathy and problems with concentration, memory, and thinking. Neuropathy is a nerve problem that causes pain, numbness, tingling, swelling, or muscle weakness in different parts of the body. It usually begins in the hands or feet and gets worse with additional cycles of treatment. Most of the time, neuropathy improves gradually and may eventually go away after treatment.

Organ issues

Treatment might cause your kidneys, liver, heart, and pancreas not to work as well as they should.

Pain

Tell your care team about any pain or discomfort. You might meet with a palliative care specialist or with a pain specialist to manage pain.

Palliative care

Palliative care is appropriate for anyone, regardless of age, cancer stage, or the need for other therapies. It focuses on physical, emotional, social, and spiritual needs that affect quality of life.

Radiation dermatitis

Radiation dermatitis is a common side effect of radiation therapy. It can cause the skin to change color or cause dry and itchy skin, pain, peeling, blistering, or swelling. Your health care provider can help you find the best treatment for radiation dermatitis.

Second cancers

Chemotherapy, immunotherapy, radiation therapy, and hematopoietic cell transplant can increase your risk of a future cancer. Therefore, it's very important to continue follow-up visits with your doctors.

Therapy-related toxicity

Many of the drug therapies used to treat lymphoma can be harmful to your body. You'll be closely monitored for therapy-related toxicity.

Tumor lysis syndrome

Lymphoma treatment causes cell death. In tumor lysis syndrome (TLS), waste released by dead cells builds up in the body, causing kidney damage and severe blood electrolyte disturbances. Changes in creatinine, lactic acid, uric acid, phosphorus, potassium, and calcium levels can be a sign of TLS. TLS can be life-threatening.

Weight gain

Weight gain is a side effect of high-dose steroids. This can be uncomfortable and cause distress. It's important to maintain muscle mass. Find a physical activity you enjoy. Ask your care team what can be done to help manage weight gain.

Key points

- Supportive care is health care that relieves symptoms caused by treatment and improves quality of life. Supportive care is always given.
- All lymphoma treatments can cause unwanted health issues called side effects. Side effects depend on many factors. These factors include the drug type and dose, length of treatment, and the person.
- Some side effects are very rare. Ask your care team what to expect.
- Tell your care team about any new or worsening symptoms.
- During and after treatment, your health will be monitored for side effects and the return of follicular lymphoma.

Questions to ask

- Who will coordinate my care?
- Who should I call when I have questions or notice changes in my condition?
- How long should I wait if I notice changes in my condition?
- What should I do on weekends and other non-office hours?
- Will my care team be able to communicate with the emergency department or urgent care team?

What's next?

The next chapter explains how classic follicular lymphoma is staged and treated.

5

Classic follicular lymphoma

Treatment for classic follicular lymphoma (cFL) is based on cancer stage. Often, treatment can wait until you have symptoms. Together, you and your care team will choose a treatment plan that's best for you.

Follicular lymphoma staging

Cancer staging is used to reflect prognosis and to help guide treatment decisions. Prognosis is the likely course your lymphoma will take. In follicular lymphoma (FL), your age, the number and location of lymph nodes affected by lymphoma, blood test results, and other factors play a role in prognosis. In addition, treatment decisions are based on histology and the results of FL biomarker and genetic tests. Histology is the overall appearance and the size, shape, and type of cells.

There are different kinds of staging systems. The Lugano Modification of Ann Arbor Staging System is used for FL. Your care team may explain your cancer stage in different ways than described next.

In general, FL stages are as follows:

- **Stage 1 (limited)** – Disease found in 1 lymph node or a group of nearby lymph nodes.
- **Stage 2 (limited)** – Disease found in 2 or more lymph node groups on the same side of the diaphragm.
- **Stage 2 bulky** – Areas of lymphoma that measure 7.5 centimeters (cm) or larger. Bulky disease can be limited or advanced.
- **Stage 3 (advanced)** – Disease found in lymph nodes above and below the diaphragm on the same side of the body, or disease found in nodes above the diaphragm and in the spleen.
- **Stage 4 (advanced)** – Disease has spread outside the lymphatic system to other parts of the body.

Lymph node regions are based on the Ann Arbor Staging System

Adapted from: Lymph_node_regions.jpg: https://commons.wikimedia.org/wiki/File:Lymph_node_regions.svg

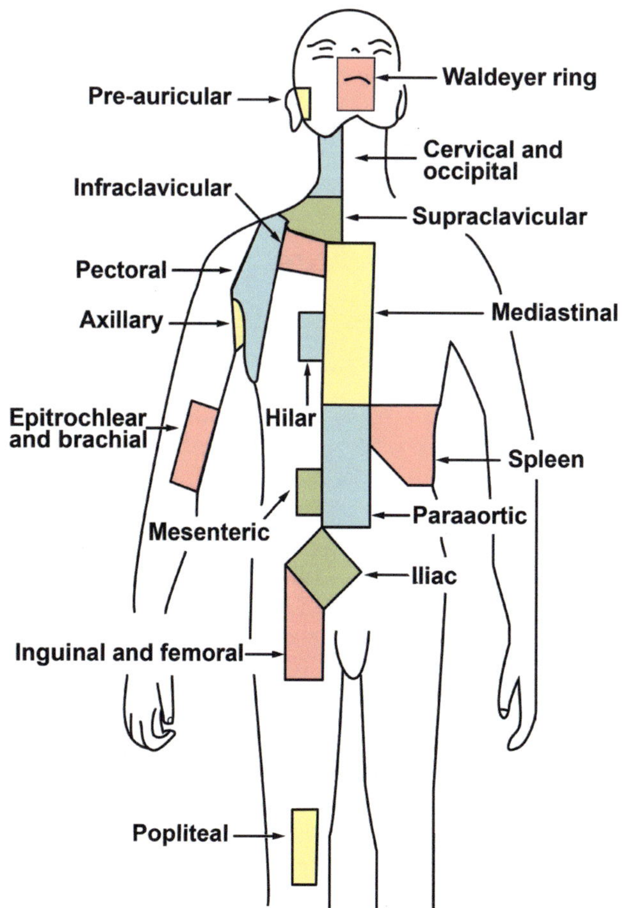

Stages 1 and 2 (limited)

Stage 1 or contiguous stage 2

In stage 1, lymphoma is found in 1 lymph node. In contiguous stage 2, lymphoma is found in lymph node groups next to one another.

For stage 1 or contiguous stage 2 disease, involved-site radiation therapy (ISRT) is the most appropriate treatment in most cases.

Other options include:

- ISRT with CD20-targeting monoclonal antibody therapy. Other systemic therapy might be added as found in **Guide 3**.
- CD20-targeting monoclonal antibody therapy (rituximab or obinutuzumab) with or without systemic therapy. Obinutuzumab isn't used by itself as a single agent. For systemic therapy options, see **Guide 3**.

Non-contiguous stage 2

Non-contiguous stage 2 disease is found in 2 or more lymph node groups on the same side of the diaphragm. Treatment options include CD20-targeting monoclonal antibody therapy. Other systemic therapy and/or radiation therapy might be added. Observation might be an option in some cases. For systemic therapy options, see **Guide 3**.

Guide 3
First-line systemic therapy options (in alphabetical order)

Preferred therapies	• Bendamustine plus Obinutuzumab or Rituximab • CHOP (Cyclophosphamide, Doxorubicin, Vincristine, and Prednisone) plus Obinutuzumab or Rituximab • CVP (Cyclophosphamide, Vincristine, and Prednisone) plus Obinutuzumab or Rituximab • Lenalidomide plus Rituximab • Rituximab
Other recommended therapies	• Lenalidomide plus Obinutuzumab

Note: An FDA-approved biosimilar might be used in place of rituximab. Extended (maintenance) therapy might be rituximab or obinutuzumab.

Treatment response

- For a complete response or partial response, observation and follow-up care are recommended.
- For no response or disease progression, see the next section called "Stages 3 and 4 (advanced)".
- For FL that has transformed into diffuse large B-cell lymphoma, read *Chapter 7: Transformed follicular lymphoma*.

> **When you are going through treatment that's difficult, remember it's about the cancer. Don't let the side effects of treatment become your focus!"**

Stage 2 follicular lymphoma

In stage 2 follicular lymphoma, cancer is found in 2 or more lymph node groups on the same side of the diaphragm.

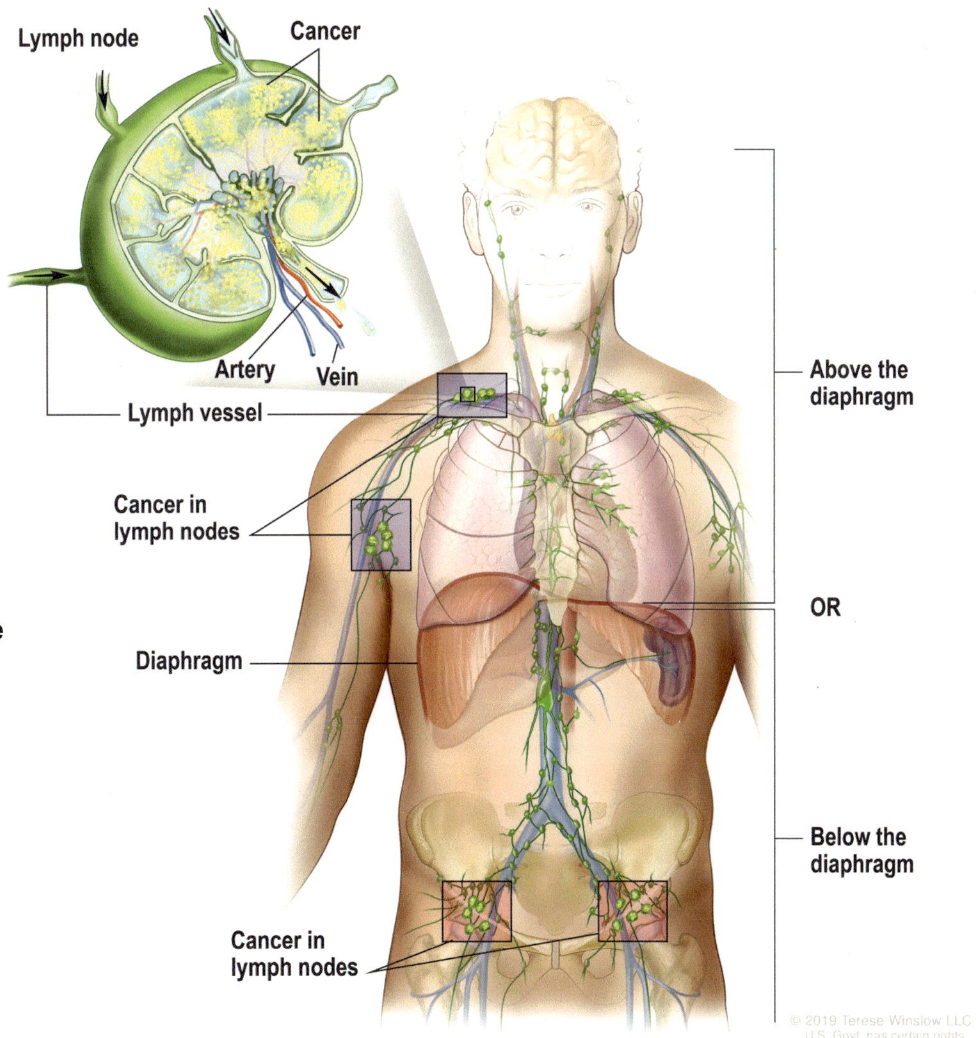

Stages 3 and 4 (advanced)

Stage 3 disease is found in lymph nodes on both sides of the diaphragm or in lymph nodes above the diaphragm and in the spleen.

Stage 4 disease is found in various areas outside the lymph nodes. This is called extranodal disease.

Observation

Your care team might wait to start treatment until certain signs or symptoms appear. This is called observation, active surveillance, or watch and wait. During this time, you'll have a physical exam, and lab tests every 3 to 6 months for 5 years and then every year afterward. You'll also have CT imaging scans with contrast every 6 months. After 2 years, you'll have a CT once a year. These CT scans are used for monitoring people who don't have symptoms. It looks for changes in your lymphoma.

Stage 3 follicular lymphoma

In stage 3 follicular lymphoma, cancer is found in lymph node groups above and below the diaphragm on the same side of the body or cancer is found in lymph nodes above the diaphragm and in the spleen.

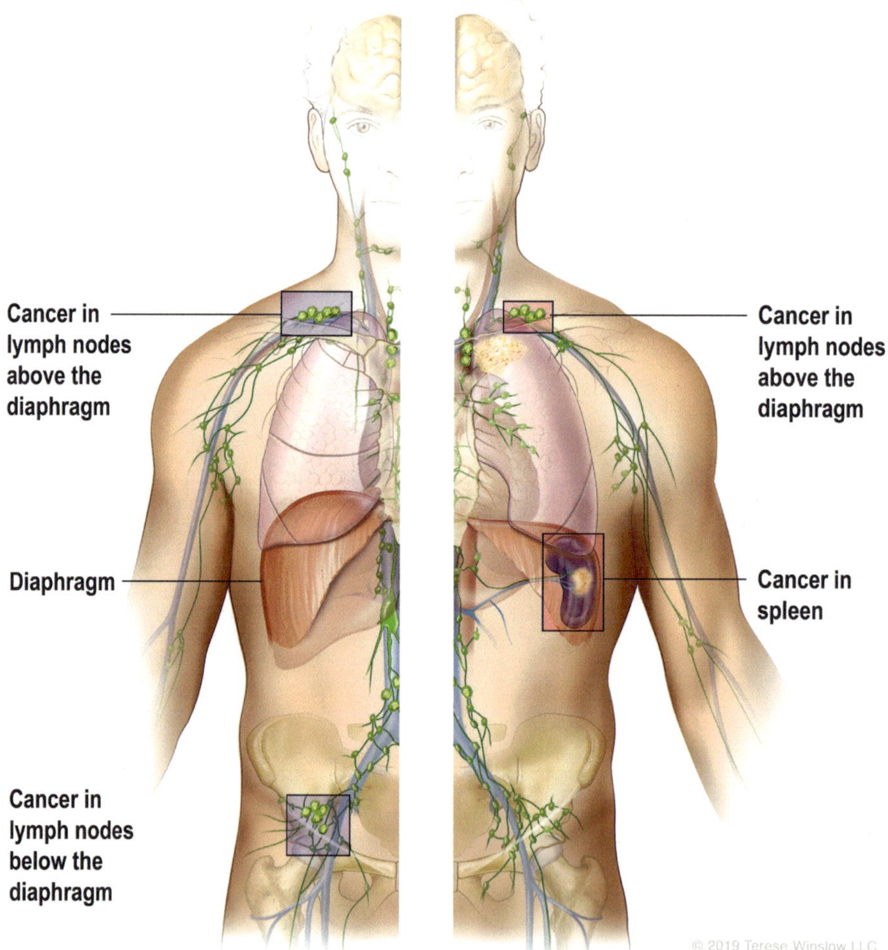

When to begin treatment

Most people with FL don't have symptoms when starting treatment. Treatment will likely start for any of the following:

- B symptoms (such as fever, night sweats, fatigue, and weight loss)
- Threatened end-organ function (damage occurring in major organs fed by the circulatory system, such as the heart, kidneys, brain, and eyes)
- Low red blood cell count (cytopenia) not caused by FL
- Bulky disease or high tumor burden as defined by Groupe d'Etude des Lymphomes Folliculaires (GELF) criteria
- Steady or rapid disease progression
- You want to start treatment
- Growth of cancer in lymph nodes, called progressive lymphadenopathy

Treatment may include systemic therapy, a clinical trial, or involved-site radiation therapy (ISRT).

First-line therapy

First-line systemic therapy is the first set of drug treatment given. For a list of first-line therapy options, see **Guide 3**.

Second-line therapy

Second-line therapy is the next set of drug treatment given. See **Guide 4**.

Guide 4
Second-line systemic therapy options (in alphabetical order)

Preferred therapies	• Bendamustine plus Obinutuzumab or Rituximab (not recommended if you had bendamustine before) • CHOP plus Obinutuzumab or Rituximab • CVP plus Obinutuzumab or Rituximab • Lenalidomide plus Rituximab plus Epcoritamab-bysp • Lenalidomide plus Rituximab plus Tafasitamab-cxix • Rituximab (if older or unwell)
Other recommended therapies	• Lenalidomide (if not candidate for CD2-targeting mAb therapy) • Lenalidomide plus Obinutuzumab or Rituximab • Obinutuzumab • Rituximab

Note: An FDA-approved biosimilar might be used in place of rituximab. Extended (maintenance) therapy might be rituximab or obinutuzumab.

Third-line therapy

If FL returns or doesn't respond to treatment, a different second-line systemic therapy will be given. After multiple lines of systemic therapy, bispecific antibody therapy or CAR T-cell therapy might be given. See **Guide 5**.

Treatment response

Imaging tests, such as PET/CT (preferred) or CT scan with contrast, will look at how the lymphoma responded to treatment and where any lymphoma might remain.

- **For a complete response (CR)**, you'll likely enter observation with follow-up care. You might have extended (maintenance) therapy.
- **For a partial response (PR)**, you might continue with your current therapy or switch to a different one.
- **For no response or disease progression**, you may have another biopsy and another round of systemic therapy with different agents (drugs) or a clinical trial. If you had 3 or more lines systemic therapy, then bispecific antibody therapy or CAR T-cell therapy might be given.
- **For FL that has transformed into diffuse large B-cell lymphoma**, see *Chapter 7: Transformed follicular lymphoma*.

Guide 5
Third- and next-line systemic therapy options (in alphabetical order)

Preferred therapies (T-cell therapy)	Bispecific antibody therapy • Epcoritamab-bysp • Mosunetuzumab-axgb
	Chimeric antigen receptor (CAR) T-cell therapy • Axicabtagene ciloleucel (CD19-directed) • Lisocabtagene maraleucel (CD19-directed) • Tisagenlecleucel (CD19-directed)
Other recommended therapies	• BTK inhibitor (BTKi) which is Zanubrutinib plus Obinutuzumab • Loncastuximab tesirine-lpyl plus Rituximab
Therapies used in certain cases	A hematopoietic cell transplant (HCT)

Note: Second-line therapies not used before might be given.

Follow-up care

After treatment, you'll be monitored with the following tests for signs and symptoms that lymphoma has returned.

- Physical exam, and lab tests every 3 to 6 months for 5 years and then every year afterward, or as needed.
- CT scan with contrast every 6 months. After 2 years, you'll have 1 CT scan a year. CT scans are used for monitoring people who don't have symptoms. They look for changes in your lymphoma.

Relapse or disease progression

Relapse is the return of lymphoma. The goal of treatment is to achieve remission again. A relapse may or may not be serious. It's possible to have multiple relapses and multiple remissions. For people with FL that relapses after more than 2 therapies, a significant number are alive at 5 years. Depending on the pace of tumor growth and the location and size of the tumor, you might not need immediate treatment.

Disease progression is when the cancer in your lymph nodes grows. Relapse and disease progression can happen without causing symptoms.

Most people with FL don't have symptoms when starting treatment. Treatment will likely start for any of the following reasons:

- B symptoms (such as fever, night sweats, fatigue, and weight loss)
- Threatened end-organ function (damage occurring in major organs) fed by the circulatory system, such as the heart, kidneys, brain, and eyes)
- A low red blood cell count (cytopenia) not related to FL
- Bulky disease or high tumor burden as defined by GELF criteria
- Steady or rapid disease progression
- You want to start treatment
- Growth of cancer in lymph nodes, called progressive lymphadenopathy

A PET/CT scan might be done before treatment is started. Treatment options include systemic therapy, clinical trial, or involved-site radiation therapy (ISRT). The goal of treatment is to achieve another remission.

Follicular lymphoma can go through long periods of remission followed by relapses. FL can also regress, or get smaller, on its own without treatment. This isn't completely understood but it's not uncommon for FL to fluctuate in size.

Key points

- Follicular lymphoma (FL) forms in and is mostly limited to the lymph nodes. However, it can be found outside the lymph nodes in areas such as bone marrow or blood.
- Treatment options include radiation therapy, systemic (drug) therapy, or a clinical trial. The goal of treatment is remission.
- Since FL is often a slow-growing disease, your care team might wait until symptoms appear before starting treatment. This is called observation, active surveillance, or watch and wait. You'll have blood and imaging tests during this time.
- Most people with FL don't have symptoms when starting treatment. This is because FL can grow or change and not cause any symptoms.
- FL often goes through periods of remission and relapse. When FL relapses or progresses, a different systemic therapy is given.
- FL can get smaller on its own without treatment. This isn't completely understood, but it's not uncommon for FL to fluctuate in size.

Questions to ask

- Is the lymphoma contiguous or noncontiguous?
- Do you think we should start treatment now or wait and why?
- What treatment do you recommend and why?
- What treatment do you think I might need after this one or down the road?
- Do you recommend a clinical trial?

What's next?

The next chapter explains how pediatric-type follicular lymphoma in adults is staged and treated.

6

Adult pediatric-type follicular lymphoma

Pediatric-type follicular lymphoma (PTFL) usually occurs in children but can also occur in adults. PTFL is stage 1 or 2. If it's stage 3 or 4, then it's not PTFL. Treatment is usually surgery to remove the tumor.

People with follicular lymphoma should seek treatment at cancer centers experienced in this type of cancer.

Testing and staging

Pediatric-type follicular lymphoma (PTFL) usually occurs in children but can also occur in adults. PTFL is stage 1 or 2 and is often found in lymph nodes in the head and neck region or sometimes the groin area. If your tumor is stage 3 or 4, then it isn't PTFL. Tumor testing will look for certain PTFL biomarkers and genetic changes. A PET/CT scan and bone marrow biopsy might be done before treatment is started.

The Lugano Modification of Ann Arbor Staging System is used for FL. In general, stages are as follows:

- **Stage 1** – Disease found in 1 lymph node or a group of nearby lymph nodes.
- **Stage 2** – Disease found in 2 or more lymph node groups on the same side of the diaphragm.
- **Stage 3** – Disease found in lymph nodes above and below the diaphragm on the same side of the body, or disease found in nodes above the diaphragm and in the spleen.
- **Stage 4** – Disease has spread outside the lymphatic system to other parts of the body.

Treatment

PTFL has an excellent prognosis and sometimes requires no treatment other than surgery to remove the tumor. Other options include radiation therapy to the tumor area or RCHOP chemoimmunotherapy. RCHOP is rituximab, cyclophosphamide, doxorubicin, vincristine, and prednisone.

After treatment, you'll enter observation and follow-up care to monitor for the return of cancer. Follow-up care includes regular physical exams, blood tests, and CT scans.

Key points

- Pediatric-type follicular lymphoma (PTFL) usually occurs in children but can also occur in adults.
- PTFL is stage 1 or 2. If it's stage 3 or 4, then it isn't PTFL.
- Stage 1 disease is found in 1 lymph node or a group of nearby lymph nodes.
- Stage 2 disease is found in 2 or more lymph node groups on the same side of the diaphragm.
- PTFL has an excellent prognosis and sometimes requires no treatment other than surgery to remove the tumor (preferred). Radiation therapy or chemoimmunotherapy might be given.
- After treatment, you'll enter observation and follow-up care to monitor for the return of cancer.
- Follow-up care includes regular physical exams, blood tests, and CT scans.

Questions to ask

- Is the lymphoma stage 1 or 2? How does the stage affect treatment options?
- What tests do I need before starting treatment?
- What treatment do you recommend and why?
- What can I expect from treatment?
- How long will treatment take?

What's next?

The next chapter provides treatment options for follicular lymphoma that transforms into diffuse large B-cell lymphoma (DLBCL). This can happen before, during, or after treatment.

7

Transformed follicular lymphoma

Follicular lymphoma (FL) can transform into a more aggressive lymphoma called diffuse large B-cell lymphoma (DLBCL). This means your slow-growing FL has turned into a large-cell, fast-growing lymphoma. Treatment is chemoimmunotherapy. Radiation therapy might be added.

Overview

Follicular lymphoma (FL) can transform into diffuse large B-cell lymphoma (DLBCL). This can occur before, during, or after treatment. In DLBCL, large-cell, fast-dividing tumors are commonly found in lymph nodes, spleen, liver, bone marrow, or other tissues and organs. The risk of transformation into DLBCL is very low. However, transformed FL is very serious.

Certain gene rearrangements or chromosome changes can be found in DLBCL. In gene rearrangements, part of a gene on a chromosome has broken off and attached itself to a gene on a different chromosome. Fluorescence in situ hybridization (FISH) is done to look for gene rearrangements.

- *MYC*, *BCL2*, and *BCL6* gene rearrangements are found in DLBCL.
- High-grade B-cell lymphomas (HGBLs) have mutations, gene rearrangements like *MYC*, or other high-risk features.

For more information on treatment for DLCBL and HGBLs, read *NCCN Guidelines for Patients: Diffuse Large B-Cell Lymphomas*, available at NCCN.org/patientguidelines and on the NCCN Patient Guides for Cancer app.

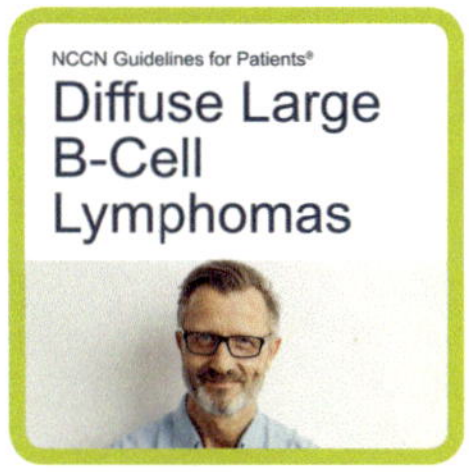

After little or no therapy

If FL changes into DLBCL after little or no therapy, then it's treated with a clinical trial or chemoimmunotherapy. Radiation therapy might be used. The goal of treatment is remission.

Preferred chemoimmunotherapy for people who can tolerate intense chemoimmunotherapy:

- RCHOP consists of rituximab, cyclophosphamide, doxorubicin, vincristine, and prednisone.
- Pola-R-CHP consists of polatuzumab vedotin-piiq, rituximab, cyclophosphamide, doxorubicin, and prednisone.

Other possible chemoimmunotherapy options include:

- DA-EPOCH-R is dose-adjusted etoposide, prednisone, vincristine, cyclophosphamide, doxorubicin, and rituximab.
- RCDOP is rituximab, cyclophosphamide, liposomal doxorubicin (Doxil), vincristine, and prednisone.

- RCEOP is rituximab, cyclophosphamide, etoposide, vincristine, and prednisone.
- RGCVP is rituximab, gemcitabine (Gemzar or Infugem), cyclophosphamide, vincristine, and prednisone.
- R-mini-CHOP and its variations for people who can't have intense chemoimmunotherapy.

Treatment response

After treatment, you'll have imaging (PET/CT) and lab tests to see if any lymphoma remains.

- In a complete response (CR) or complete remission, no lymphoma remains. Observation or a clinical trial are options. If disease relapses, you'll have a biopsy before treatment.
- If there's a partial response (PR), then you'll be given CD19-targeting CAR T-cell therapy. Other systemic therapies are possible.
- If your disease doesn't respond to treatment or has progressed, then you'll be given CD19-targeting CAR T-cell therapy. Other systemic therapies are possible.

After multiple lines of therapy

If FL changed into DLBCL after multiple lines of therapy, then treatment options include:

- Clinical trial
- Systemic therapy. Options are based on what you were treated with before, your situation, and other factors. A type of radiation therapy called involved-site radiation therapy (ISRT) might be added to treat lymphoma located in a small region or 1 area of your body.
- ISRT
- Best supportive care (improves quality of life and relieves discomfort)

The goal of treatment is remission. If a hematopoietic cell transplant (HCT) is being considered, it's usually decided early in treatment planning because having HCT affects future treatment options. Certain treatments aren't recommended before or after HCT. Bispecific antibody therapy can be given after cellular therapy (HCT or CAR T-cell therapy).

If lymphoma returns or doesn't respond to treatment, another systemic therapy will be given. After multiple lines of systemic therapy, CD19-targeting CAR T-cell therapy or bispecific antibody therapy might be given.

Treatment response

After treatment, you'll have imaging (PET/CT scan) and lab tests to see if any lymphoma remains.

Complete response

In a complete response (CR), or remission, no lymphoma remains. You might enter observation. An autologous (self) or allogeneic (donor) hemopoietic cell transplant (HCT) may be an option. After treatment, you'll enter surveillance and be monitored for relapse.

Partial response

In a partial response (PR), treatment options are based on the types of treatment you had before. Options listed below depend on your individual situation:

- CD19-targeting CAR T-cell therapy (preferred, if not given before)
- Allogeneic HCT in some cases. ISRT might be added if not given before.
- ISRT (if not given before and disease is in a small region or 1 area of your body)
- Observation with follow-up tests

Relapse

If disease relapses, you'll have a biopsy before treatment. Treatment might include a clinical trial, a systemic therapy not used before, ISRT, CD19-targeting CAR T-cell therapy, bispecific antibody therapy, or best supportive care. In best supportive care, the focus is improving quality of life and relieving discomfort.

No response or disease progresses

When disease progresses during treatment or doesn't respond to any treatment after multiple lines of therapy, the focus is on best supportive care.

Key points

- Follicular lymphoma (FL) can transform into diffuse large B-cell lymphoma (DLBCL). This means your slow-growing FL has turned into a large-celled, fast-growing, aggressive lymphoma.
- The goal of treatment for transformed FL is remission.
- If FL changed into DLBCL after little or no treatment, then it's treated with chemoimmunotherapy, such as RCHOP or Pola-R-CHP. Radiation therapy might be given.
- If FL changed into DLBCL after multiple lines of therapy, then the treatment recommendations include a clinical trial, systemic therapy, radiation therapy, or best supportive care. In best supportive care, the focus is improving quality of life and relieving discomfort.
- A hematopoietic cell transplant (HCT) might be an option in some cases after multiple lines of systemic therapy. If an HCT is being considered, it's usually decided early in treatment planning.
- The order of treatment matters.
- Bispecific antibody therapy is an option before or after HCT or CD19-targeting CAR T-cell therapy.

Questions to ask

- Where do you think we should start with treatment?
- What order of treatments are you considering and why?
- How many rounds of treatment do you think I'll need?
- Are you planning for a hematopoietic cell transplant (HCT) in the future?
- Am I a candidate for a clinical trial?

What's next?

The next chapter provides information about resources and where you can get support.

We want your feedback!

Our goal is to provide helpful and easy-to-understand information on cancer. Take our survey to let us know what we got right and what we could do better. NCCN.org/patients/feedback

8

Other resources

Want to learn more? Here's how you can get additional help.

What else to know

This guide helps you know your options so you can make informed decisions and improve your cancer care. But it's not the only resource that you have.

Ask for as much information and help as you need. Many people are interested in learning more about:

- Finding an oncologist who's an expert in treating lymphoma
- Making treatment decisions, including waiting to start treatment
- The details of treatment and possible side effects
- Getting financial help
- Coping with stress of having follicular lymphoma

What else to do

Your health care center can help you with next steps. It often has on-site resources to help meet your needs and find answers to your questions. Health care centers can also inform you of resources in your community.

In addition to help from your providers, the resources listed in the next section provide support for many people like yourself.

Where to get help

Look through the list below and visit the provided websites to learn more about these organizations.

AnCan Foundation
ancan.org

Blood & Marrow Transplant Information Network
bmtinfonet.org

Blood Cancer United
bloodcancerunited.org

Cancer*Care*
cancercare.org

Cancer Hope Network
cancerhopenetwork.org

HealthTree Foundation
healthtree.org

Imerman Angels
imermanangels.org

Lymphoma Research Foundation
lymphoma.org

National Bone Marrow Transplant Link (nbmtLINK)
nbmtlink.org

NMDP
nmdp.org

PAN Foundation
panfoundation.org

Triage Cancer
triagecancer.org

Questions to ask

- Who can I talk to about help with housing, food, and other basic needs?
- What help is available for transportation, childcare, and home care?
- What other services are available to me and my caregivers?
- How can I connect with others and build a support system?
- Who can I talk to if I don't feel safe at home, at work, or in my neighborhood?

"I want people to know 2 things. One, there are experts out there who treat your type of cancer. And, two, there are resources and support available to you. Don't be afraid to ask your doctor questions or ask your friends for help."

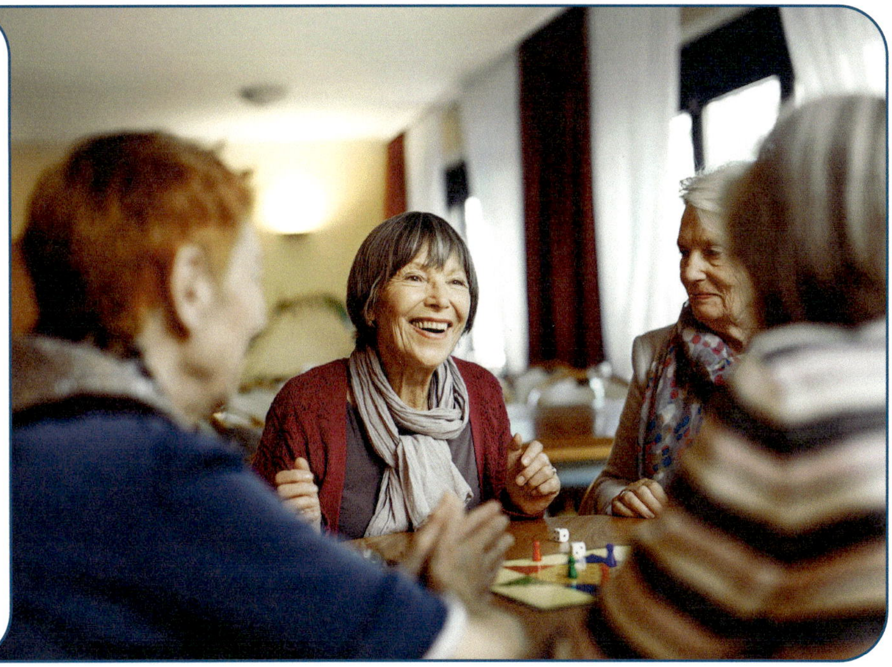

Words to know

allogeneic hematopoietic cell transplant (allogeneic HCT)
Cancer treatment that destroys your bone marrow then rebuilds it with healthy donor cells.

autologous hematopoietic cell transplant (autologous HCT)
Cancer treatment that destroys your bone marrow then rebuilds it with your healthy stem cells. Also called high-dose therapy with autologous stem cell rescue (HDT/ASCR).

best supportive care
Treatment to improve quality of life and relieve discomfort.

biomarker testing
A lab test of any molecule in your body that can be measured to assess your health. Also called molecular testing.

biopsy
A procedure that removes fluid or tissue samples to be tested for a disease.

biosimilar
A drug that's almost identical to a drug made by another company. It's been approved by the U.S. FDA and must be used in the exact same way and at the same dose as the other drug.

bone marrow
The sponge-like tissue in the center of most bones.

bone marrow aspiration
A procedure that removes a liquid bone marrow sample to test for a disease.

bone marrow biopsy
A procedure that removes bone and solid bone marrow samples to test for a disease.

chromosome
The structures within cells that contain coded instructions for cell behavior.

clinical trial
A type of research that assesses health tests or treatments.

complete response (CR)
No signs of lymphoma are found. Also called complete remission.

computed tomography (CT)
A test that uses x-rays from many angles to make a picture of the inside of the body.

contrast
A substance put into your body to make clearer pictures during imaging tests.

deoxyribonucleic acid (DNA)
A chain of chemicals in cells that contains coded instructions for making and controlling cells.

flow cytometry
A lab test of substances on the surface of cells to identify the type of cells present.

fluorescence in situ hybridization (FISH)
A lab test that uses special dyes to look for abnormal chromosomes and genes.

gene
A set of coded instructions in cells for making new cells and controlling how cells behave.

hematopathologist
A doctor who specializes in the study of blood diseases and cancers using a microscope.

hematopoietic cell transplant (HCT)
A cancer treatment that replaces abnormal blood stem cells with healthy cells. Also called stem cell transplant (SCT) or bone marrow transplant (BMT).

histology
The study of tissues and cells under a microscope.

imaging test
A test that makes pictures (images) of the inside of the body.

immune system
The body's natural defense against infection and disease.

immunohistochemistry (IHC)
A lab test of cancer cells to find specific cell traits involved in abnormal cell growth.

immunophenotyping
A lab test that detects the type of cells present based on the cells' surface proteins.

involved-site radiation therapy (ISRT)
Radiation therapy that treats cancer found in a small region or 1 area of the body.

karyotype
Lab test that makes a map of chromosomes to find defects.

lactate dehydrogenase (LDH)
A protein in blood that helps to make energy in cells.

lymph
A clear fluid containing white blood cells.

lymph node
A small, bean-shaped, disease-fighting structure.

lymphadenopathy
Lymph nodes that are abnormal in size or consistency.

lymphatic system
A germ-fighting network of tissues and organs that includes the bone marrow, spleen, thymus, lymph nodes, and lymphatic vessels. Part of the immune system.

lymphedema
Swelling in the body due to a buildup of fluid called lymph.

lymphocyte
A type of white blood cell that's part of the immune system.

magnetic resonance imaging (MRI)
A test that uses radio waves and powerful magnets to make pictures of the inside of the body.

maintenance
The last phase of treatment used over a long period to prevent cancer from returning.

monitoring
A period of testing for changes in cancer status.

mutation
An abnormal change in the instructions within cells for making and controlling cells.

partial response (PR)
Lymphoma is still present but has reduced in size.

pathologist
A doctor who's an expert in testing cells and tissue to find disease.

peripheral blood (PB)
Blood that circulates throughout the body.

platelet (PLT)
A type of blood cell that helps control bleeding. Also called a thrombocyte.

positron emission tomography (PET)
A test that uses radioactive material to see the shape and function of body parts.

prognosis
The likely course a disease will take.

radiation therapy (RT)
A treatment that uses high-energy rays.

recovery
A period of time without treatment to allow blood cell counts to return to normal.

recurrence
Return of cancer after a cancer-free period.

red blood cell (RBC)
A type of blood cell that carries oxygen from the lungs to the rest of the body. Also called an erythrocyte.

refractory cancer
A cancer that doesn't improve with treatment.

relapse
The return or worsening of cancer after a period of improvement.

remission
Minor or no signs of disease.

side effect
An unhealthy or unpleasant physical or emotional response to treatment.

spleen
An organ that's part of the lymphatic system. The spleen makes lymphocytes, filters the blood, stores blood cells, and destroys old blood cells. It's located on the left side of the abdomen near the stomach.

supportive care
Treatment for the symptoms or health conditions caused by cancer or cancer treatment. Also sometimes called palliative care or best supportive care.

translocation
A switching of parts between 2 chromosomes.

tumor lysis syndrome (TLS)
A condition caused when waste released by dead cells isn't quickly cleared out of your body.

white blood cell (WBC)
A type of blood cell that helps fight infections in the body. Also called a leukocyte.

NCCN Contributors

This patient guide is based on the NCCN Clinical Practice Guidelines in Oncology (NCCN Guidelines®) for B-Cell Lymphomas, Version 4.2026. It was adapted, reviewed, and published with help from the following people:

Dorothy A. Shead, MS
Senior Director
Patient Information Operations

Tanya Fischer, MEd, MSLIS
Senior Medical Writer

Lisa Diehl
Production Layout Artist

The NCCN Clinical Practice Guidelines in Oncology (NCCN Guidelines®) for B-Cell Lymphomas, Version 4.2026, were developed by the following NCCN Panel Members:

Andrew D. Zelenetz, MD, PhD/Chair
Memorial Sloan Kettering Cancer Center

*Leo I. Gordon, MD/Vice Chair
Robert H. Lurie Comprehensive Cancer Center of Northwestern University

Jeremy S. Abramson, MD, MMSc
Mass General Cancer Center

Ranjana H. Advani, MD
Stanford Cancer Institute

Alaa Altahan, MD
St. Jude Children's Research Hospital/ The University of Tennessee Health Science Center

Babis Andreadis, MD, MSCE
UCSF Helen Diller Family Comprehensive Cancer Center

Nancy L. Bartlett, MD
Siteman Cancer Center at Barnes-Jewish Hospital and Washington University School of Medicine

*L. Elizabeth Budde, MD, PhD
City of Hope National Medical Center

Paolo F. Caimi, MD
Case Comprehensive Cancer Center/ University Hospitals Seidman Cancer Center and Cleveland Clinic Taussig Cancer Institute

Sven DeVos, MD, PhD
UCLA Jonsson Comprehensive Cancer Center

Bhagirathbhai Dholaria, MD
Vanderbilt-Ingram Cancer Center

Luis E. Fayad, MD
The University of Texas MD Anderson Cancer Center

Sameh Gaballa, MD
Moffitt Cancer Center

*Thomas M. Habermann, MD
Mayo Clinic Comprehensive Cancer Center

*Francisco Hernandez-Ilizaliturri, MD
Roswell Park Comprehensive Cancer Center

Boyu Hu, MD
Huntsman Cancer Institute at the University of Utah

Manali Kamdar, MD
University of Colorado Cancer Center

Yasmin Karimi, MD
University of Michigan Rogel Cancer Center

Christopher R. Kelsey, MD
Duke Cancer Institute

Rebecca King, MD
Mayo Clinic Comprehensive Cancer Center

Justin Kline, MD
The UChicago Medicine Comprehensive Cancer Center

Susan Krivacic, MPAff
Patient advocate

Ann S. LaCasce, MD, MMSc
Dana-Farber/Brigham and Women's Cancer Center

Daniel Landsburg, MD
Abramson Cancer Center at the University of Pennsylvania

Megan Lim, MD, PhD
Memorial Sloan Kettering Cancer Center

Marcus Messmer, MD
Fox Chase Cancer Center

Priyanka Pophali, MD
University of Wisconsin Carbone Cancer Center

Rachel Rabinovitch, MD
University of Colorado Cancer Center

Praveen Ramakrishnan, MD, MS
UT Southwestern Simmons Comprehensive Cancer Center

Erin Reid, MD
UC San Diego Moores Cancer Center

Peter Riedell, MD
The UChicago Medicine Comprehensive Cancer Center

Kenneth B. Roberts, MD
Yale Cancer Center/Smilow Cancer Hospital

Aditi Saha, MD
O'Neal Comprehensive Cancer Center at UAB

*Naoyuki G. Saito, MD, PhD
Indiana University Melvin and Bren Simon Comprehensive Cancer Center

Yazeed Sawalha, MD
The Ohio State University Comprehensive Cancer Center - James Cancer Hospital and Solove Research Institute

Stephen D. Smith, MD
Fred Hutchinson Cancer Center

Lode J. Swinnen, MBChB, MD
Johns Hopkins Kimmel Cancer Center

Joseph Tuscano, MD
UC Davis Comprehensive Cancer Center

Julie M. Vose, MD, MBA
Fred & Pamela Buffett Cancer Center

NCCN

Mary Dwyer, MS
Senior Director, Clinical Operations

Hema Sundar, PhD
Senior Manager, Global Clinical Content

* Reviewed this patient guide. For disclosures, visit NCCN.org/disclosures.

NCCN Cancer Centers

For contact information, visit NCCN.org/cancercenters.

Abramson Cancer Center
at the University of Pennsylvania
Philadelphia, Pennsylvania

Case Comprehensive Cancer Center/
University Hospitals Seidman Cancer Center and
Cleveland Clinic Taussig Cancer Institute
Cleveland, Ohio

City of Hope National Medical Center
Duarte, California

Dana-Farber Cancer Institute
Boston, Massachusetts

Duke Cancer Institute
Durham, North Carolina

Fox Chase Cancer Center
Philadelphia, Pennsylvania

Fred & Pamela Buffett Cancer Center
Omaha, Nebraska

Fred Hutchinson Cancer Center
Seattle, Washington

Huntsman Cancer Institute at the University of Utah
Salt Lake City, Utah

Indiana University Melvin and Bren Simon
Comprehensive Cancer Center
Indianapolis, Indiana

Johns Hopkins Kimmel Cancer Center
Baltimore, Maryland

Mass General Brigham Cancer Institute
Boston, Massachusetts

Mayo Clinic Comprehensive Cancer Center
Phoenix/Scottsdale, Arizona
Jacksonville, Florida
Rochester, Minnesota

Memorial Sloan Kettering Cancer Center
New York, New York

Moffitt Cancer Center
Tampa, Florida

O'Neal Comprehensive Cancer Center at UAB
Birmingham, Alabama

Robert H. Lurie Comprehensive Cancer Center
of Northwestern University
Chicago, Illinois

Roswell Park Comprehensive Cancer Center
Buffalo, New York

Siteman Cancer Center at Barnes-Jewish Hospital
and WashU Medicine
St. Louis, Missouri

St. Jude Children's Research Hospital/
The University of Tennessee Health Science Center
Memphis, Tennessee

Stanford Cancer Institute
Stanford, California

The Ohio State University Comprehensive Cancer Center -
James Cancer Hospital and Solove Research Institute
Columbus, Ohio

The UChicago Medicine Comprehensive Cancer Center
Chicago, Illinois

The University of Texas MD Anderson Cancer Center
Houston, Texas

UC Davis Comprehensive Cancer Center
Sacramento, California

UC San Diego Moores Cancer Center
La Jolla, California

UCLA Jonsson Comprehensive Cancer Center
Los Angeles, California

UCSF Helen Diller Family Comprehensive Cancer Center
San Francisco, California

University of Colorado Cancer Center
Aurora, Colorado

University of Michigan Rogel Cancer Center
Ann Arbor, Michigan

University of Wisconsin Carbone Cancer Center
Madison, Wisconsin

UT Southwestern Simmons
Comprehensive Cancer Center
Dallas, Texas

Vanderbilt-Ingram Cancer Center
Nashville, Tennessee

Yale Cancer Center/Smilow Cancer Hospital
New Haven, Connecticut

Index

Made in the USA
Monee, IL
15 September 2026

63296729R00040